THE PERIMENOPAUSE RESET

THE PERIMENOPAUSE RESET

28 DAYS TO ENERGIZE YOUR BODY, SHED WEIGHT, AND FIND PEACE WITH GOD

BY
JENNIFER PFLEGHAAR, DO, ABOIM

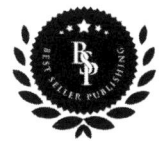

Copyright © 2025 by Jennifer Pfleghaar, DO, ABOIM

All rights reserved. No part of this book may be used or reproduced in any manner whatsoever without prior written consent of the author, except as provided by the United States of America copyright law.

Published by Best Seller Publishing®, St. Augustine, FL
Best Seller Publishing® is a registered trademark.
Printed in the United States of America.

ISBN: 978-1-969338-91-5

This publication is designed to provide accurate and authoritative information with regard to the subject matter covered. It is sold with the understanding that the publisher is not engaged in rendering legal, accounting, or other professional advice. If legal advice or other expert assistance is required, the services of a competent professional should be sought. The opinions expressed by the author in this book are not endorsed by Best Seller Publishing® and are the sole responsibility of the author rendering the opinion.

For more information, please write:
Best Seller Publishing®
1775 US-1 #1070
St. Augustine, FL 32084
or call 1 (626) 765-9750

Visit us online at: www.BestSellerPublishing.org

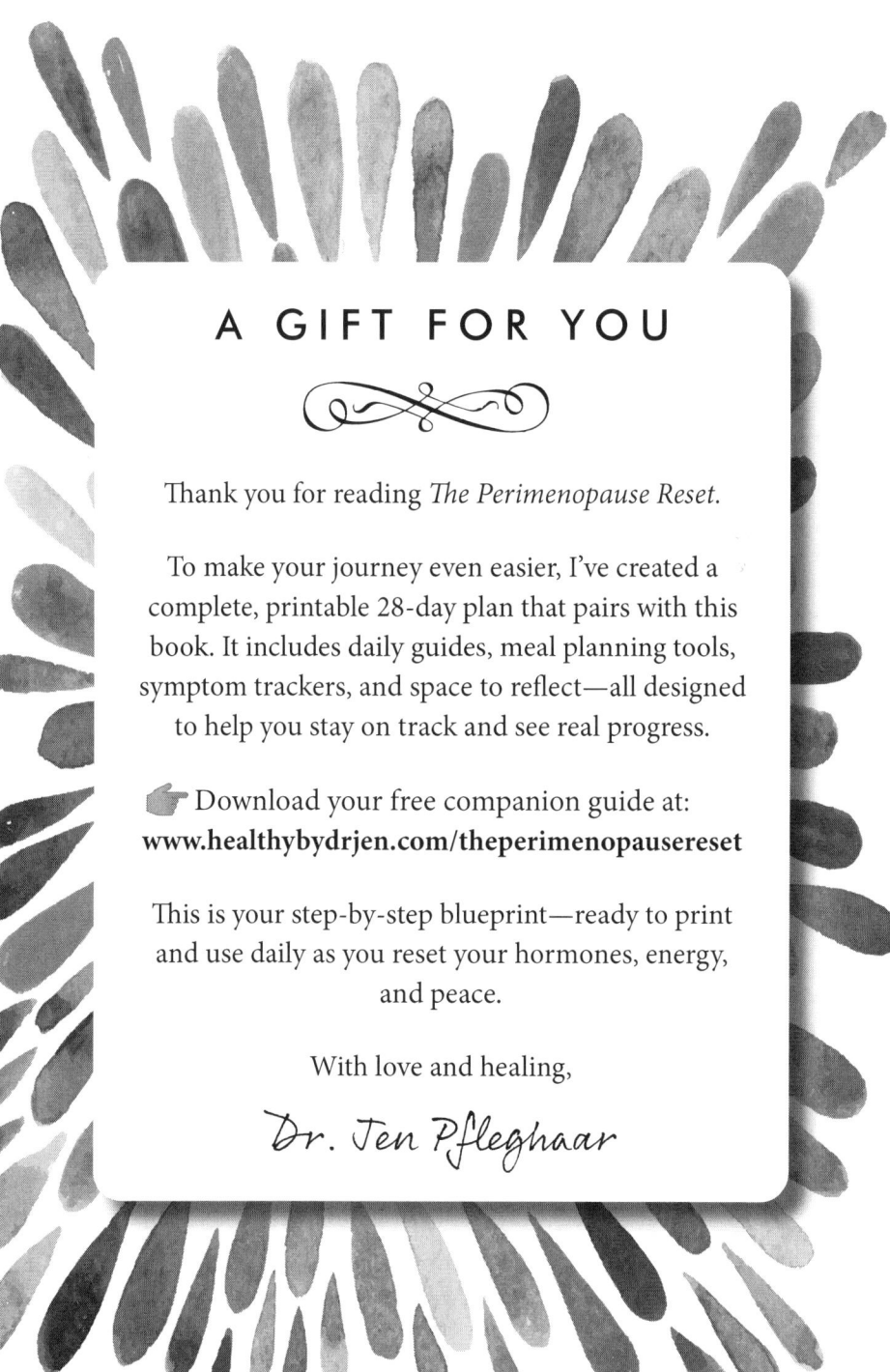

A GIFT FOR YOU

Thank you for reading *The Perimenopause Reset*.

To make your journey even easier, I've created a complete, printable 28-day plan that pairs with this book. It includes daily guides, meal planning tools, symptom trackers, and space to reflect—all designed to help you stay on track and see real progress.

👉 Download your free companion guide at:
www.healthybydrjen.com/theperimenopausereset

This is your step-by-step blueprint—ready to print and use daily as you reset your hormones, energy, and peace.

With love and healing,

Dr. Jen Pfleghaar

Table of Contents

Medical Disclaimer xi

Advance Praise xiii

Foreword xvii

Introduction: A Journey to Healing 1

    Understanding the Menstrual Cycle and Perimenopause 5

PART 1: ENVIRONMENT 13

Chapter 1: Cleanse Your Home 15

    Make Your Environment a Healthy Place! 15

    The Environmental Threat to Hormone Health 16

    What Are Endocrine Disruptors? 17

    Phthalates: Softening Plastic, Disrupting Hormones 17

    Parabens: Preservatives with Estrogenic Effects 17

    Bisphenol A (BPA): A Common Disruptor in Plastics 18

    Heavy Metals: Interference with Hormonal and
Metabolic Pathways 18

    How Endocrine Disruptors Affect Mood, Metabolism,
and Overall Health 19

    Reducing Exposure to Endocrine Disruptors 19

Chapter 2: Connect with Better Products 21

    Fourteen Ways to Connect to a Cleaner Environment 23

    Connecting with Your Circadian Rhythm to
Optimize Hormones 28

    How Your Circadian Rhythm Influences Hormones 28

    Steps to Sync Your Circadian Rhythm 29

Chapter 3: Cultivate a Healthy Habitat 33

    Cultivate a Mold-Free Environment 34

    What Are Mycotoxins? 34

    Hormone Effects of Mycotoxins 36

    Preventing Mold in Your Home 38

    Cultivate a Sweet Sleep Environment 39

    Smart Sleep Supplementation 43

PART 2: BODY 47

Chapter 4: Cleanse from Within 51

    What Are GMO Crops? 52

    The Gut-Hormone Axis in Perimenopause 55

    Why Gluten Can Lead to Intestinal Permeability 57

    Time to Cleanse, Connect, and Cultivate with Liver Detoxification 61

Chapter 5: Connect to Your Endocrine Signals 73

    Connect to Fasting for Your Health 74

    What About Coffee on an Empty Stomach? 80

    Benefits of Continuous Glucose Monitors 82

    Peptides for Perimenopause: What About GLP-1s? 91

Chapter 6: Cultivate Strength 95

    Hormonal Shifts: A Factory for Muscle Health 96

    Building Muscle During Perimenopause 103

    Cultivate a Smart Nutrition Plan to Address
    Hormonal Shifts 115

    Peptides in Perimenopause 122

PART 3: SPIRIT **127**

Chapter 7: Cleanse: Release to Restore 131

    Surround Yourself with Good Things 131

    Cleanse Your Environment of Toxicity and Negativity 138

Chapter 8: Connect to Jesus 141

    Yoga: Deceitful Peace and Hidden Darkness 144

    Stress Reduction with Meditation and Breathwork:
    Natural Support for Perimenopause 145

    What About the Vagus Nerve? 148

Chapter 9: Cultivate a Deep Relationship with God 153

    Reading the Bible 154

    Connect with Truth: Planting a Seed of Connection
    with God 158

    Spiritual Warfare 160

Chapter 10: Cycle Syncing 163

    Diet: Eating for Your Cycle 164

    How Estrogen and Progesterone Affect Blood Sugar 168

    The Menstrual Cycle and Exercise: Sync Your Workouts 168

PART 4: 28-DAY PLAN AND DEVOTIONAL **175**

    Your 28-Day Plan to Energize Your Body, Shed Weight,
    and Find Peace with God 177

    Your Daily Cycle Day Devotional 181

    Conclusion 213

    Acknowledgments 217

References and Resources 219

    Chapter 1 219

    Chapter 2 220

    Chapter 3 220

    Chapter 4 221

    Chapter 5 222

    Chapter 6 223

    Chapter 7 225

    Chapter 8 225

    Chapter 10 226

Index 231

About the Author 233

Medical Disclaimer

This book is intended for educational and informational purposes only. Although the author is a licensed medical doctor, the content herein is not intended to serve as a substitute for individualized medical advice, diagnosis, or treatment.

Discussions related to nutrition, supplements, hormone therapy, lab testing, or lifestyle strategies are general in nature and may not be appropriate for every individual. Readers are strongly encouraged to consult their personal healthcare provider before making any changes to medications, beginning new supplements, adjusting hormone therapy, or interpreting laboratory results.

The author and publisher disclaim any liability for outcomes resulting from the use or misuse of the information presented. Reliance on any information provided in this book is solely at the reader's discretion and risk.

Advance Praise

"Dr. Jenny Pfleghaar brings together the best of integrative medicine and unwavering faith to guide women through the often-overlooked journey of perimenopause. Her book is a compassionate, evidence-based, and spiritually nourishing guide that empowers women to heal at the root and reclaim vibrant hormonal health."

—Dr. Jill Carnahan, MD
Medical Director, Flatiron Functional Medicine
Author of *Unexpected: Finding Resilience through Functional Medicine, Science, and Faith*

"This book by Dr. Jen flows out of her passion to help women thrive in physical health and spiritual vitality. I have seen this to be the focus in both her personal life and her professional life. I encourage you to read it if you desire that to be true of your life as well."

—Dennis T. Ditto
Senior Pastor

"*The Perimenopause Reset* is the empowering, faith-rooted guide I wish every woman had during midlife. Dr. Pfleghaar beautifully combines science, integrative medicine, and spiritual support to help women address the root causes of perimenopausal symptoms, and not just survive this season, but truly thrive. Her compassionate, practical approach will leave you feeling informed, inspired, and seen."

—Izabella Wentz, PharmD
Author of *Hashimoto's Protocol*

"Truth-filled, empowering, and practical. This book is a must-read for women who want to take control of their health through the perimenopause transition."

—Ashley Goin

Owner, Innate Health Chiropractic

"What can I say, this book is a breath of fresh air.

"Perimenopause is such a delicate balancing act for many women, and oftentimes we have no clue where to start with getting our health back on track.

"This book is so informative with life-changing information that can be easily implemented into your daily routine. Dr. Pfleghaar is bringing to light that health is more than just following protocols and procedures, but it's also about your spiritual well-being and being rooted in your identity in Christ.

"I love how this book intertwines health with scripture and encourages women that we don't need to feel tired, anxious, and stressed as we enter a new season of life. Dr. Pfleghaar emphasizes that as we are striving to regain our health, we also need to rest in Jesus and remember that our bodies are wonderfully created to heal."

—Rickie Neill

Healed and thriving, by God's grace and Dr. Jen's care

"In The Perimenopause Reset, Dr. Jen is trailblazing; letting Jesus lead her and boldly proclaiming the gospel through everything she does, including medicine. Testifying of His goodness, Dr. Jen offers a comprehensive integrative approach (sans new age nonsense) to optimal health for women navigating change. She gets what so many miss; for we know that true healing only comes from The Healer."

—Nicole McManus, D.C.

"*The Perimenopause Reset is a transformative and empowering guide for women navigating the often-overlooked season of perimenopause. Blending science-based medical advice with faith-driven encouragement, the book equips readers to reclaim their health by addressing environmental toxins, hormonal imbalances, and spiritual well-being. Dr. Pfleghaar's compassionate voice and personal experiences make complex topics relatable and actionable, offering a holistic 28-day plan to reset body, mind, and spirit. This book is both a deeply informative resource and a heartfelt companion for any woman seeking to thrive through perimenopause.*"

—Lori Bryant, FNTP

Director of Seeking Whole Health

"*The Perimenopause Reset: 28 Days to Energize Your Body, Shed Weight, and Find Peace with God will be so helpful in getting to the root of your hormonal issues. As a patient and friend of Dr. Jen, I'm so thankful for this resource to guide me through this unknown season of life. Dr. Jen is gifted with being able to apply scripture and medicine together.*"

—Sheila Schlatter

Canal Junction Farm

"*As an integrative pediatrician, I've witnessed how perimenopause can catch mothers completely off guard—draining our energy, stealing our sleep, and shifting our very sense of self. In* The Perimenopause Reset, *Dr. Jen Pfleghaar delivers exactly what women need: a compassionate, faith-based, science-backed guide to reclaiming our bodies and our joy. This isn't just a book—it's a blueprint for transformation, empowering women to thrive through perimenopause and change the trajectory of their health for decades to come.*"

—Dr. Elisa Song

Integrative pediatrician and bestselling author of *Healthy Kids, Happy Kids*

"Dr. Jen's book is a transformative guide, masterfully blending cutting-edge science with spiritual wisdom, filling a vital gap in modern medicine. Her practical protocols and authentic, uplifting message empower women to take charge of their healing through hormonal transitions. This must-read offers lasting hope for those seeking to align body, mind, and spirit, breaking free from the roller coaster of conventional healthcare. Dr. Jen's work shines as a beacon of light, guiding women toward their maximum potential with deep, holistic healing."

—Dr. Lindsey Miuccio, DAOM, DAC, Lac

Dr. Jen has paved a path to empowering women during a natural life transition—not with drugs and sadness—but with the glory of God and the wonderment that nature cures. To embrace the beauty of this change in a woman's life with such natural grace is a gift everyone can embrace. Thank you for leading us to a higher level of self-caring.

—Robin Rose MD
Holistic Family Medicine, author of *RENOLOGY Peptides - a definitive guide to kidney success with bioregulator peptides*

FOREWORD

The Perimenopause Reset by Dr. Jennifer Pfleghaar is a unique look at a time in a woman's life that may be one of her most challenging. Commonly, women's hormones become imbalanced, and she may develop symptoms of anxiety, irritability, insomnia, mood swings, depression, and hot flashes. It is also the same time that if she has children, they are maturing and may have challenges of their own.

This book focuses on a biblical perspective to women's health. We are born perfect in the eyes of the Lord. Unfortunately, due to stress, environmental toxins, and an unhealthy diet, the body usually develops hormonal imbalances that can occur anytime in a woman's life but are common at the ages of 35–55. This text provides a myriad of key concepts and solutions to help the body heal and detoxify, from a natural viewpoint.

In addition, one of the most frustrating symptoms of perimenopause is weight gain. Dr. Pfleghaar explores many new and interesting ways to help the body obtain and maintain the perfect weight.

One of the greatest truths of this book, which sets it apart from many other books on women's hormones, is that the author has a special understanding of the concept that in order to be healthy, you have to be physically healthy, emotionally healthy, and spiritually healthy. It is only by God's grace and our cultivating a closer relationship with the Lord that we able to achieve optimal health. God has given Dr. Pfleghaar an exceptional gift to help women at this time in their lives. This book is a must read for all women, no matter their age.

Pamela W. Smith, M.D., MPH, MS
Author of What You Must Know About
Women's Hormones 1st and 2nd Editions

INTRODUCTION

A Journey to Healing

*For wisdom will enter your heart, and
knowledge will be pleasant to your soul.*

—Proverbs 2:10 (NIV)

This book is about knowledge. My prayer is that this knowledge will be pleasant to your soul.

What I've seen in nearly two decades of practicing medicine is that patients suffer—not just from disease, but from a lack of knowledge, especially knowledge about how to prevent disease in the first place.

Women are often ignored in medicine. Maybe you're feeling "off," but you don't know why. Your periods might be getting shorter or longer. You may feel more irritable the week before your cycle. You're acting a little more emotional, maybe even overwhelmed or stressed—and wondering what's going on.

Welcome to perimenopause.

The good news? You don't have to struggle through this. You can thrive through it.

In my practice, I noticed a pattern—so many women entering the perimenopause stage came in asking for help. They weren't okay. They felt dismissed, alone, and frustrated. Some were offered antidepressants or told that weight gain and fatigue were just "normal." They felt gaslit by their conventional medicine doctors.

But here's the truth: that's not normal. And it's not your only option.

In this book, we're going to get to the root causes. You can lose weight, gain energy, and feel like yourself again.

I know what this feels like personally. I started noticing that I was more impatient with my kids, even yelling sometimes the week before my period. My cycle had shortened to 26 days. I recognized that perimenopause had begun. I tightened my blood sugar control, focused on estrogen detox, and supported natural progesterone production. The difference was incredible—I felt like myself again. Actually, I felt even better than I had in my 20s!

So how did I know how to regulate my cycle? Let's go back to the beginning.

One of my first memories involving medicine was when my grandpa was rushed to UPMC hospital in Pittsburgh. I was nine years old. After his bypass surgery, I remember listening to the doctor explain things, and I knew in that moment—I wanted to become a doctor.

In high school, I was diagnosed with hypothyroidism after they found a thyroid nodule. I started treatment with medication, and my fascination with medicine only deepened. I remember asking God in college if medicine was the path He had for me. He answered yes, and I kept going.

During my first year of medical school, the thyroid nodule had grown. I had surgery over Christmas break after finishing my finals. Praise God, it wasn't cancer—but the surgeon told me I had Hashimoto's thyroiditis and that there was nothing I could do about it.

But I wasn't convinced. I struggled to feel better afterward. My thyroid levels were difficult to regulate, and I remember sitting in the doctor's office in tears—advocating for myself, showing published research on why adding T3 might help. At the time, I was on monotherapy (T4) and still struggling with energy difficulties. Even while being a medical student, it was still difficult to get someone to listen!

Years later, while working in an emergency room, I removed gluten from my diet and addressed SIBO (small intestinal bacterial overgrowth). For the first time, my Hashimoto's antibodies dropped to zero. That's when I knew what true healing looked like. I went on to complete a fellowship in Integrative Medicine.

Over the years, I have seen hundreds of women dealing with perimenopausal symptoms who were told by their primary care doctors, "You're just tired because you're a mom." They were handed birth control or antidepressants as a quick fix.

Let me be clear—symptoms are not just something to suppress. They're signs. God beautifully and wonderfully made our bodies. Symptoms are signals, pointing us to deeper imbalances that can be addressed. We are given symptoms to get to the root cause, not to ignore or band-aid the symptoms with medications.

Scripture:

I praise you, for I am fearfully and wonderfully made.
Wonderful are your works; my soul knows it very well.

—Psalm 139:14 (ESV)

In this book, you'll find faith-based and evidence-based solutions to help you balance your hormones, clean up your environment, understand your cycle, and reconnect with God. You'll learn how to match your diet and workouts to your cycle, and how to walk through this season with both grace and strength.

I've seen that midlife can be one of the hardest stages for women—emotionally, physically, and spiritually. Some walk through divorce or midlife crisis; others wrestle with identity or turn to New Age practices looking for healing.

You don't need that. What you need is peace—real peace. And that comes from aligning your mind, body, and spirit while keeping your eyes on Jesus.

Just like Ruth, who faced hardship and change, yet stayed faithful and trusted God, we too can walk this transition with purpose. During perimenopause, we may feel like outsiders in our own bodies, but by trusting in God and keeping our eyes on Jesus, we can come out victorious. Ruth became part of the lineage of King David—and eventually, Jesus—reminding us that God's plans are often at work in our most uncertain seasons.

Here's a summary of the most common symptoms by hormone changes during perimenopause:

- Irregular periods
- Missed periods
- Shorter or longer cycle lengths
- Increased anxiety
- Irritability
- Depression or sadness
- Brain fog and forgetfulness
- Insomnia
- Waking up in the middle of the night
- Restless sleep
- Hot flashes
- Night sweats
- Unexplained weight gain
- Bloating and water retention
- Breast tenderness
- Joint pain and muscle stiffness
- Increased headaches or migraines
- Vaginal dryness
- Decreased libido

More frequent UTIs
Leaking urine when sneezing or laughing
Thinning hair or hair loss
Drier skin
Acne breakouts
Slower digestion
More sensitivity to certain foods
Increased gas or stomach discomfort
Heart palpitations

Understanding the Menstrual Cycle and Perimenopause

One of the best ways to understand your body—and what's happening in perimenopause—is to get familiar with the rhythm of your menstrual cycle.

Each month, your body follows a carefully choreographed four-phase cycle, primarily guided by two key hormones: estrogen and progesterone. Think of it like a well-planned event. Each phase has a purpose, a mood, and a tone—like different parts of a beautifully organized party.

It all begins with menstruation—the clean-up phase when you get ready for the event. This is the quiet reset, where your body sheds the uterine lining from the previous cycle. Estrogen and progesterone are at their lowest, and it's common to feel more introverted or low energy during this time.

Then comes the follicular phase, where estrogen rises and takes center stage. This is the grand opening. Energy increases, mood lifts, and many women feel more motivated, focused, and social. Skin glows, confidence rises, and it's often a time of increased creativity and clarity.

At ovulation, the party hits its peak. Testosterone rises briefly, adding a boost of confidence, energy, and libido. Many women feel more vibrant, outgoing, and self-assured during this time.

After that, progesterone steps in during the luteal phase—like the calm host who helps wind down the celebration. If progesterone is in balance, you'll feel grounded, reflective, and ready to wind down smoothy. But if progesterone is low or stress is high, this is when emotional "guests" can act out—mood swings, bloating, anxiety and, insomnia may crash the scene. If no pregnancy occurs, the venue resets, and the cycle begins again.

This cyclical rhythm is how your body has kept time for years. But as you enter perimenopause, the pattern begins to change.

What Happens in Perimenopause?

Perimenopause is the transitional stage before menopause—often beginning in a woman's late 30s or early 40s—when hormones start to fluctuate in new and unexpected ways.

Progesterone is usually the first to decline. As levels drop, symptoms like heavier periods, increased anxiety, poor sleep, or shorter cycles can appear. Estrogen, meanwhile, becomes unpredictable. Some months it surges—leaving you wired, bloated, or irritable. Other months it's too low, resulting in fatigue, depression, or night sweats.

The once-smooth event now feels like a chaotic gathering: the playlist is off, the lights are flickering, and the mood swings through extremes without warning. It's still your body—but suddenly it's harder to manage.

When the body experiences prolonged stress—whether from work, relationships, or lack of sleep—it diverts resources to handle the emergency, pulling from progesterone to fund cortisol production. This progesterone "steal" leaves the party in even more chaos, causing insomnia, anxiety, and estrogen dominance.

BUT THE PARTY ISN'T OVER

This transition doesn't mean your cycle—or your vitality—is ending. It simply means your body is asking for a new kind of support.

With the right tools—like hormone-supportive nutrition, stress reduction, proper sleep, gentle detox, herbal support, and, when appropriate, bioidentical hormones—you can help restore peace to the system.

The rhythm may be changing, but that doesn't mean you have to feel lost. It's possible to move into this next phase of life feeling confident, energetic, and anchored.

In some cases, a trusted co-host (bioidentical progesterone) can step in to restore order. With the right approach, the transition from the monthly cycle to menopause doesn't have to feel like a chaotic, never-ending event. Instead, it can shift into a new kind of celebration—one that's calmer, more intentional, and in harmony with this new phase of life.

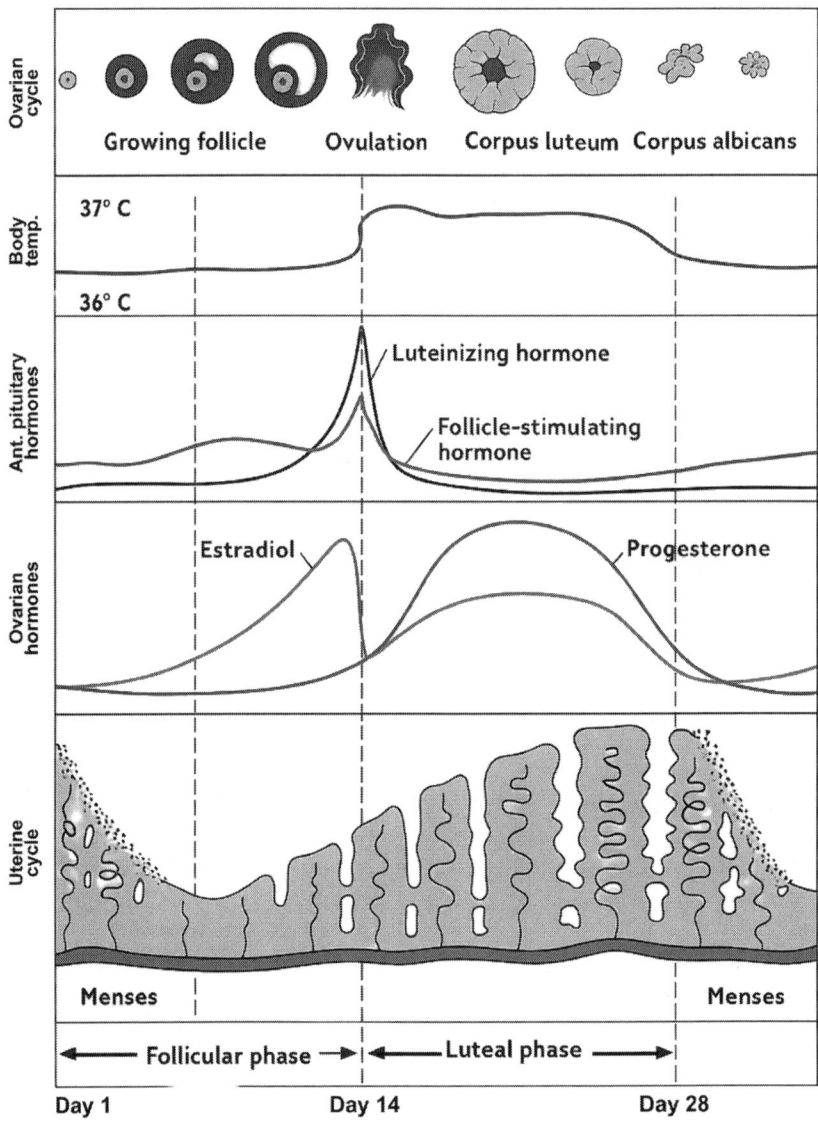

Menstrual Cycle and Hormones

HORMONE

DHEA

Function:

A steroid hormone that serves as a precursor to testosterone and estrogens, it plays a role in aging, energy levels, immune function, and mental clarity.

Primary Production Site:

Adrenal glands.

Effects on the Body:

Supports energy production, slows aging effects, enhances immune function, improves mental clarity, and helps regulate metabolism.

Imbalances & Effects:

Low levels can cause fatigue, depression, and poor immune function. High levels can lead to androgenic effects like acne and excess hair growth.

TESTOSTERONE

Function:

A crucial androgen responsible for the development of male characteristics, muscle growth, libido, bone density, red blood cell production, and overall well-being.

Primary Production Site:

Ovaries, adrenal glands.

Effects on the Body:

Promotes muscle mass, enhances strength, increases libido, maintains bone density, stimulates red blood cell production, and influences mood.

Imbalances & Effects:

Low levels cause fatigue, depression, muscle loss, and low libido. High levels can cause aggression, hair loss, and prostate issues.

HORMONE

ESTRONE (E1)

Function:

A weak estrogen primarily produced in fat cells and the adrenal glands. It can be converted into estradiol and estriol, and it plays a role in postmenopausal estrogen balance.

Primary Production Site:

Ovaries, adipose tissue.

Effects on the Body:

Regulates estrogen levels in postmenopausal women, supports bone health, and can be converted into other estrogens as needed.

Imbalances & Effects:

Higher levels linked to weight gain, breast tenderness, and possible estrogen-sensitive tissue stimulation.

ESTRADIOL (E2)

Function:

The most biologically active estrogen, essential for reproductive function, menstrual cycle regulation, cardiovascular health, and bone maintenance. It influences mood and cognitive function.

Primary Production Site:

Ovaries.

Effects on the Body:

Crucial for fertility, regulates menstrual cycles, maintains cardiovascular health, supports brain function, and modulates mood.

Imbalances & Effects:

Declines during perimenopause, leading to irregular cycles, mood swings, hot flashes, and sleep disturbances.

HORMONE

ESTRIOL (E3)

Function:

The least potent estrogen, mainly produced during pregnancy to support fetal development and maintain the uterine lining. It helps modulate estrogenic activity.

Primary Production Site:

Placenta (during pregnancy), peripheral conversion from E1.

Effects on the Body:

Plays a balancing role; supports vaginal, urinary, and skin tissue without overstimulating breast or uterine tissue.

Imbalances & Effects:

Low levels may contribute to vaginal dryness, urinary symptoms, skin thinning, and decreased tissue elasticity.

PREGNENOLONE

Function:

A precursor steroid hormone synthesized from cholesterol. It is the starting point for the synthesis of DHEA, testosterone, progesterone, and cortisol.

Primary Production Site:

Adrenal glands, gonads, brain.

Effects on the Body:

Acts as a hormonal precursor, aiding in the synthesis of sex hormones and adrenal hormones, essential for overall hormonal balance.

Imbalances & Effects:

Low levels can lead to hormone deficiencies, fatigue, and stress intolerance. High levels may lead to hormonal overproduction disorders.

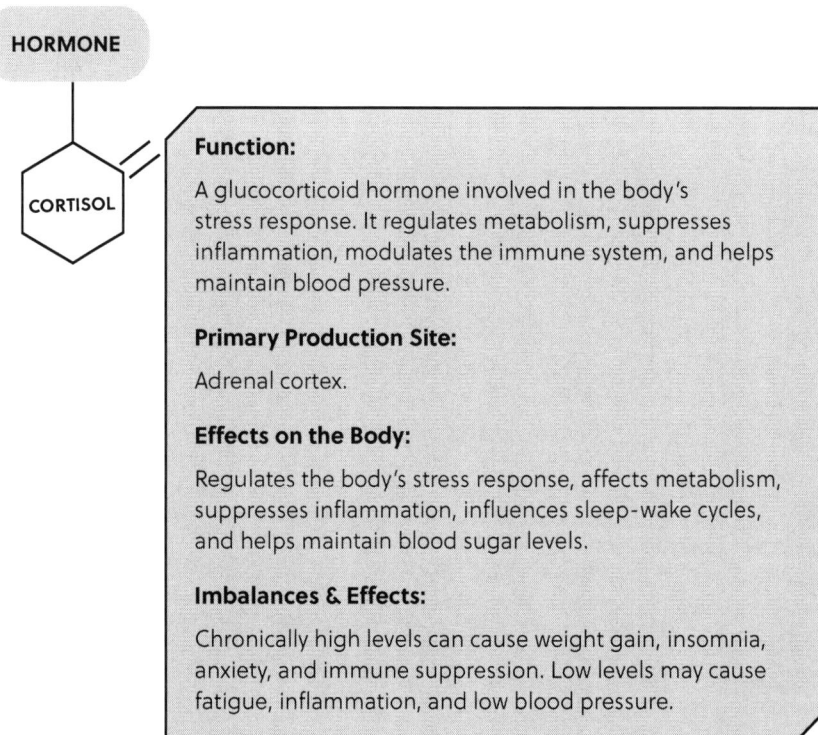

Perimenopause is a hormonal roller coaster—a season before menopause when key hormone levels fluctuate unpredictably. Navigating these changes requires working with your body, not against it. But this isn't just a physical journey—it's an emotional and spiritual one, too. When stress runs high or life feels overwhelming, it's easy to drift from our time with the Lord. Yet it's in these very moments that we need His presence the most. In this season of change, staying anchored in Jesus isn't just helpful—it's essential.

Let's begin the perimenopause reset—together.

> Rejoice always, pray without ceasing, give thanks in all circumstances; for this is the will of God in Christ Jesus for you.
>
> —1 Thessalonians 5:16–17 (NIV)

Part 1:
Environment

CHAPTER 1

Cleanse Your Home

Make Your Environment a Healthy Place!

Sue was a busy mom of two hockey-playing boys, juggling schedules and responsibilities like so many women do. She had started feeling more irritable before her cycle, noticed her periods were getting shorter, and was gaining weight—even though nothing had changed in her diet or exercise routine. When she spoke to her primary care physician, she was told she was "just depressed" and prescribed an antidepressant. Thankfully, Sue did not take that advice, declined the prescription, and came to see me instead.

We began by cleaning her environment and diet, introducing key supplements, and incorporating prayerful meditation into her daily routine. After three months, we repeated her labs. Her estrogen and progesterone were more balanced, her blood sugar had improved, and her symptoms had significantly decreased. She felt more energized, began losing weight, and—most importantly—finally felt like herself again.

Does this sound like you? If so, you are in the majority! Let's get started on the perimenopause reset.

> Cleanse me with hyssop, and I will be clean;
> wash me, and I will be whiter than snow.
>
> —Psalms 51:7 (NIV)

When I was in middle school, some of my favorite memories were made wandering the Millcreek Mall in Erie, Pennsylvania, with my friends. We'd head straight for Victoria's Secret and Bath & Body Works, sampling the latest scents and stocking up on lotions. At the time, it felt harmless and fun. We had no idea that many of those fragrances could quietly disrupt our hormones.

Every Christmas, my dad would gift me a new bottle of perfume—something I truly looked forward to. But once I learned about the impact of synthetic fragrance on the body, I gently asked him to pause the tradition. It wasn't an easy change, but when it comes to our health, sometimes the small shifts matter most. Detoxing our environment is one of the first and most powerful steps we can take toward healing.

The Environmental Threat to Hormone Health

Our hormonal health is intricately connected to the world around us. Environmental factors, including specific chemicals known as endocrine disruptors, can interfere with the body's endocrine system, affecting hormone production, metabolism, and receptor function. These chemicals—found in everyday items such as plastics, personal care products, and industrial materials—can mimic or block hormones, potentially disrupting the body's natural balance. This chapter explores how endocrine disruptors like phthalates, parabens, BPA (bisphenol A), and heavy metals impact hormone health and influence conditions related to mood, metabolism, and reproductive health.

Have you ever heated up something in a plastic container, say something like tomato sauce, and it turns the container a different color? That plastic is leaching into your food and into your body.

What Are Endocrine Disruptors?

Endocrine disruptors are chemicals that can interfere with endocrine (or hormone) systems at certain doses, leading to adverse developmental, reproductive, neurological, and immune effects.

These substances can bind to hormone receptors, mimic hormones (often estrogen), block hormone receptor sites, or interfere with the synthesis, transport, and metabolism of natural hormones. This is basically like a security officer sitting outside of your hormone receptors and not letting your hormones through the door to do their job.

Phthalates: Softening Plastic, Disrupting Hormones

Phthalates are commonly used as plasticizers in a wide range of products, from cosmetics and food packaging to medical devices and children's toys.

Research shows that phthalates can disrupt the function of androgens and estrogens. This can affect reproductive health and potentially leads to hormone-related disorders. Studies link phthalate exposure to reduced testosterone levels in men and altered reproductive development.

Animal studies have shown that phthalates impact metabolic health, and have associations with obesity and insulin resistance. In humans, prenatal phthalate exposure has been linked to reproductive abnormalities and hormonal imbalances in offspring.

Parabens: Preservatives with Estrogenic Effects

Parabens are preservatives used in cosmetics, pharmaceuticals, and foods to prevent microbial growth. Check the back of your tortillas; parabens are even added as a food preservative.

They can act as estrogen mimics, binding to estrogen receptors and potentially disrupting normal hormonal function. Research indicates that they can accumulate in human tissues, with studies finding parabens in breast tissue samples. There is growing evidence that parabens may contribute to breast cancer development due to their estrogenic effects. This means these chemicals can attach to estrogen receptors in breast tissue, mimicking natural estrogen and potentially stimulating the growth of hormone-responsive cells.

Bisphenol A (BPA): A Common Disruptor in Plastics

BPA is used in polycarbonate plastics and epoxy resins, found in water bottles, food containers, and the linings of metal cans. This potent endocrine disruptor mimics estrogen by binding to estrogen receptors. It can affect multiple hormonal pathways, including those involved in reproductive and metabolic processes.

BPA exposure has been linked to early puberty in girls, polycystic ovarian syndrome (PCOS), fertility issues, and metabolic disorders, including insulin resistance and obesity. Animal studies suggest that BPA exposure may also affect the hypothalamus, leading to altered brain development and behavioral changes.

Heavy Metals: Interference with Hormonal and Metabolic Pathways

Heavy metals such as lead, mercury, cadmium, and arsenic are environmental contaminants found in food, water, and soil. They can disrupt hormone function by binding to receptors, altering hormone production, or interfering with hormone metabolism. For example, lead exposure has been associated with changes in thyroid hormone levels, which can affect metabolism and energy balance. Mercury, on the other hand, has been shown to disrupt adrenal hormone production and interfere with the metabolism of catecholamines—important chemicals like adrenaline and noradrenaline that help regulate stress responses and cardiovascular function.

Exposure to heavy metals has been associated with a range of health issues, including impaired reproductive function, neurodevelopmental delays, and metabolic disorders. Heavy metals have also been implicated in increasing oxidative stress, which can damage endocrine tissues and disrupt hormone production.

How Endocrine Disruptors Affect Mood, Metabolism, and Overall Health

Some endocrine disruptors impact the production of neurotransmitters such as serotonin and dopamine, potentially influencing mood and behavior. BPA, for example, has been associated with increased anxiety and depression in animal studies.

Chemicals like phthalates and BPA have been linked to obesity and metabolic syndrome. They interfere with glucose metabolism, reduce insulin sensitivity, and alter fat storage, contributing to weight gain and related health issues. These compounds can weaken immune function, raise the risk of immune-related disorders, and disrupt reproductive health, leading to conditions such as PCOS, infertility, and hormone-related cancers. In perimenopause, exposure to endocrine disruptors may further compound hormonal fluctuations, worsening symptoms like weight gain, mood changes, and metabolic imbalance.

Reducing Exposure to Endocrine Disruptors

Given the widespread presence of endocrine disruptors in our environment, minimizing exposure is essential for supporting hormone health. Choosing BPA-free products, limiting plastic use, and opting for natural personal care items can help reduce exposure to these chemicals.

Check out more helpful videos on how to clean out your home and what to swap on my YouTube channel:

https://www.youtube.com/@integrativedrmom

Chapter Key Takeaways:

- Your environment can silently affect your hormones
- Endocrine disruptors can affect hormone health
- Start small by making simple changes like buying natural, non-toxic products

CHAPTER 2

Connect with Better Products

For my yoke is easy, and my burden is light.
—Matthew 11:30 (NIV)

I had a nonstick wok that I loved for one specific dish I would cook for my family: homemade chicken nuggets fried in beef tallow. It was a great pan for frying, but I knew it wasn't good for our health. Perfluorooctanoic acid (PFOA), found in nonstick coatings, can disrupt your hormones and hormone receptors. Worse yet, they are called forever chemicals because they aren't broken down in the environment or in your body. A study on firefighters who had significant exposure from their fireproof suits revealed that only bloodletting (giving blood) was able to decrease their bodies' burden of PFOAs.

I had gotten rid of every nonstick pan we owned ... except for that one. It worked so well. Sigh, I threw it out. I knew I had to.

We need to unburden ourselves with fewer toxic products in our house, just as we give our burdens to Jesus. We need to take the environmental burdens out of our home, connecting with better products. I get it: just like my favorite wok, it was hard to let go, but my body thanks me for it. So many of us are troubled by this reality and the truth is, we don't need to be. Toss the toxins and connect with a healthier life.

What Are Forever Chemicals?

Perfluorooctanoic acid (PFOA), a type of per- and polyfluoroalkyl substance (PFAS), is known to interfere with the endocrine system, particularly affecting hormone function and receptors. Research indicates that PFOA can disrupt thyroid hormone levels, potentially leading to hypothyroidism. This disruption occurs because PFOA can mimic fatty acids, allowing it to bind to proteins involved in hormone transport and metabolism, thereby altering normal hormonal activities.

In a study involving Australian firefighters, researchers explored methods to reduce elevated PFAS levels resulting from occupational exposure. The study divided participants into three groups: one group donated plasma every six weeks, a second donated whole blood every 12 weeks, and the control group did not donate. Results showed that plasma donation was the most effective intervention, reducing mean serum perfluorooctane sulfonate (PFOS) levels by 2.9 ng/mL, compared to a 1.1 ng/mL reduction with blood donation. Similar reductions were observed for other PFAS compounds, including PFOA. This suggests that regular plasma donations may help decrease PFAS levels in individuals with high exposure.

Fourteen Ways to Connect to a Cleaner Environment

Each of these steps helps connect you to a cleaner, healthier environment, reducing your exposure to everyday toxins.

1. Plastic Containers: Replace with glass or stainless steel to avoid BPA and other plasticizers.
2. Non-Stick Cookware: Opt for stainless steel or cast iron to avoid chemicals like PFOA and PTFE.
3. Air Fresheners: Use natural alternatives like essential oils, or open windows for ventilation.
4. Processed Foods: Avoid foods with artificial preservatives, colors, and flavors.
5. Personal Care Products with Phthalates/Parabens: Choose phthalate-free, paraben-free options for lotions, shampoos, and cosmetics.
6. Synthetic Fragrances: Choose fragrance-free or naturally scented (essential oil) products.
7. Tap Water: Filter tap water to remove chemicals and heavy metals. Reverse osmosis is a great method, but make sure to add back in electrolytes.
8. Detergents and Dish Soap: Swap for natural, fragrance-free options to reduce exposure to harsh chemicals.
9. Household Cleaners: Replace with eco-friendly cleaners without chlorine, ammonia, or bleach. Vinegar and baking soda can work great.
10. Fast Food Packaging: Avoid fast food and food packaged in coated paper to reduce exposure to PFAS (often used as grease-proofing). Bring your own to-go containers to restaurants.
11. Mattresses and Bedding: Opt for organic or chemical-free options to reduce flame retardant and volatile organic compounds (VOC) exposure.
12. Electronics: Minimize exposure to blue light and EMF radiation by unplugging electronics when not in use, especially in the bedroom.

13. Leave your shoes at the door! Don't wear shoes inside the home. They can track toxins into your home. Instead, keep slippers for use inside the house.
14. Check inactive ingredients in your medications and ask about them, if you receive them from the pharmacy. Medications can contain food dyes, gluten, and toxic fillers.

Medication Ingredients to Watch Out for!

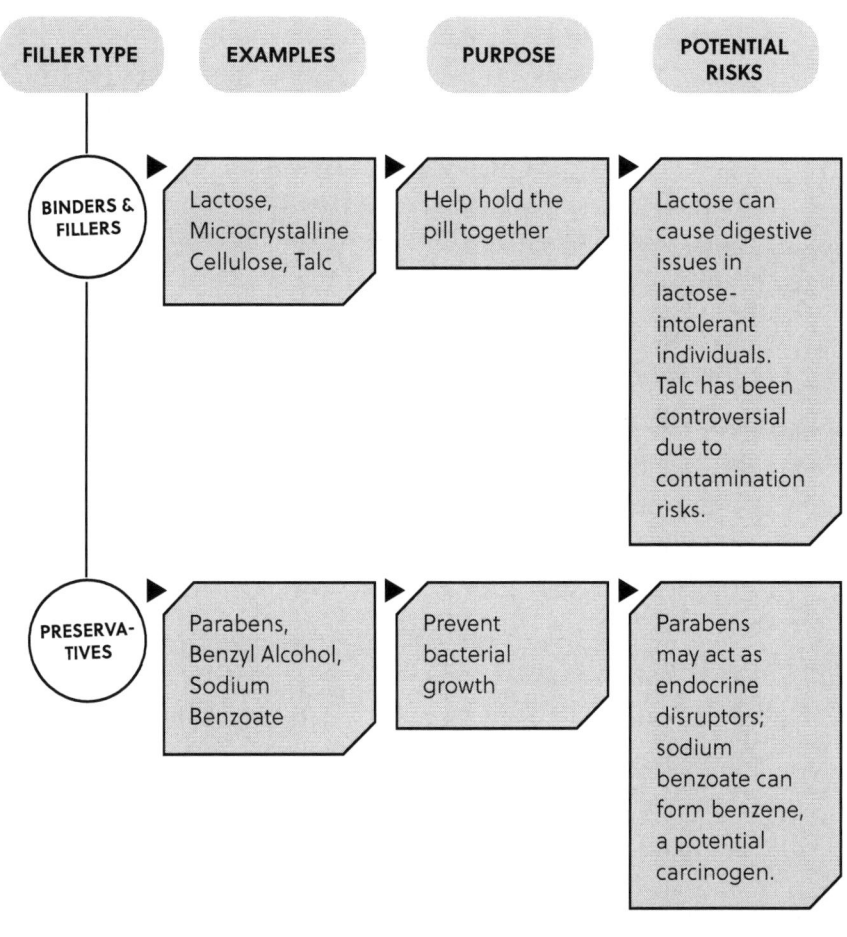

FILLER TYPE	EXAMPLES	PURPOSE	POTENTIAL RISKS
BINDERS & FILLERS	Lactose, Microcrystalline Cellulose, Talc	Help hold the pill together	Lactose can cause digestive issues in lactose-intolerant individuals. Talc has been controversial due to contamination risks.
PRESERVATIVES	Parabens, Benzyl Alcohol, Sodium Benzoate	Prevent bacterial growth	Parabens may act as endocrine disruptors; sodium benzoate can form benzene, a potential carcinogen.

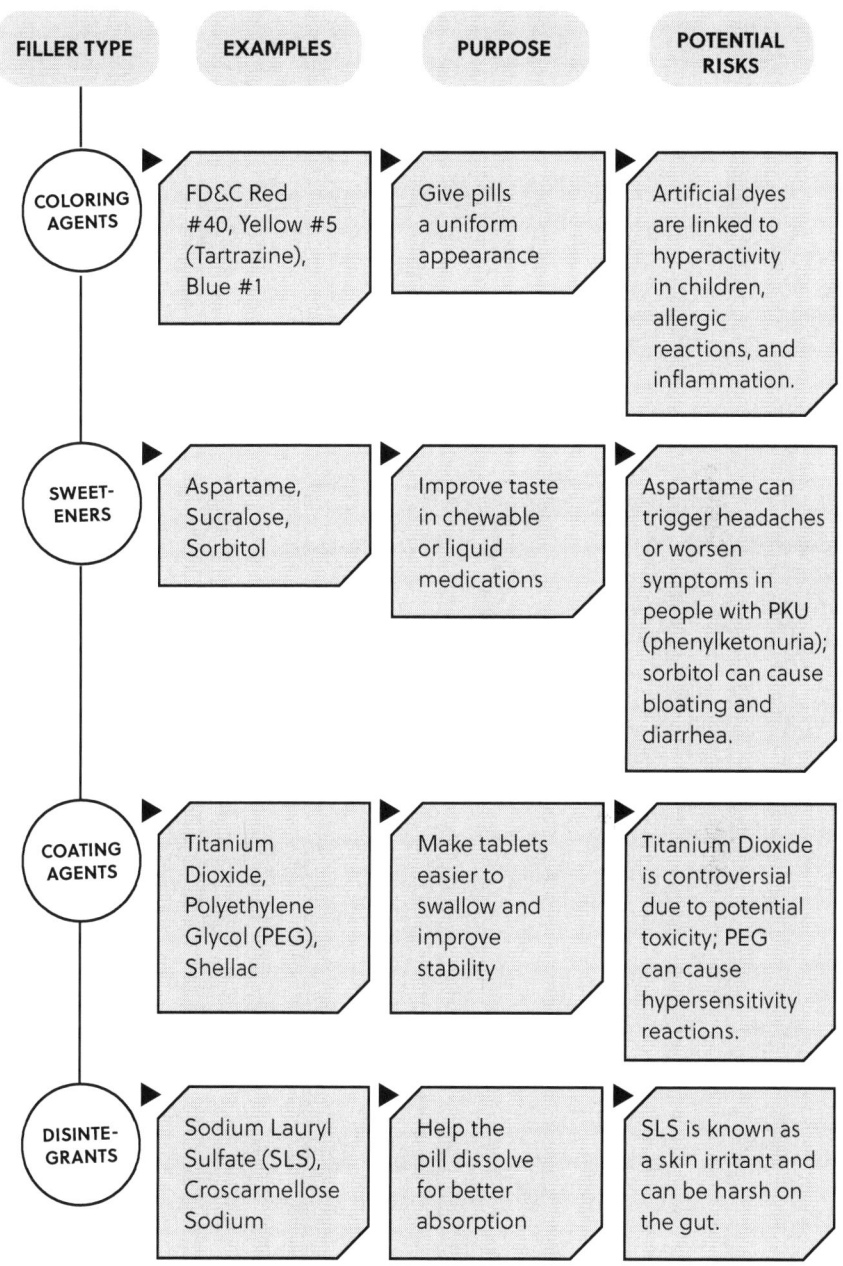

FILLER TYPE	EXAMPLES	PURPOSE	POTENTIAL RISKS
COLORING AGENTS	FD&C Red #40, Yellow #5 (Tartrazine), Blue #1	Give pills a uniform appearance	Artificial dyes are linked to hyperactivity in children, allergic reactions, and inflammation.
SWEETENERS	Aspartame, Sucralose, Sorbitol	Improve taste in chewable or liquid medications	Aspartame can trigger headaches or worsen symptoms in people with PKU (phenylketonuria); sorbitol can cause bloating and diarrhea.
COATING AGENTS	Titanium Dioxide, Polyethylene Glycol (PEG), Shellac	Make tablets easier to swallow and improve stability	Titanium Dioxide is controversial due to potential toxicity; PEG can cause hypersensitivity reactions.
DISINTEGRANTS	Sodium Lauryl Sulfate (SLS), Croscarmellose Sodium	Help the pill dissolve for better absorption	SLS is known as a skin irritant and can be harsh on the gut.

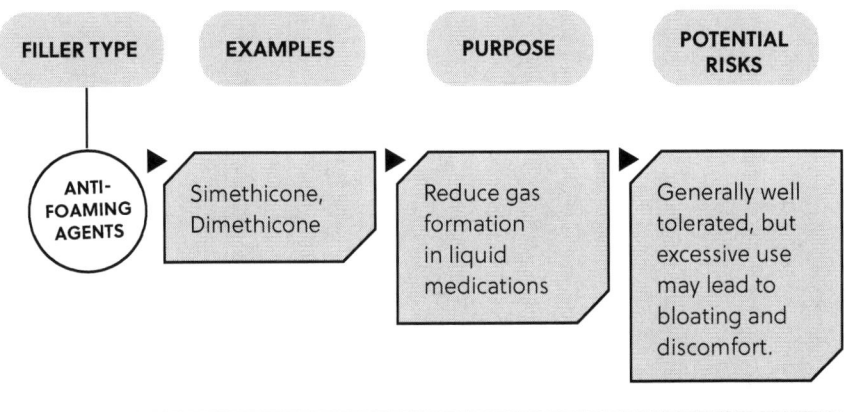

Cleanse, Connect, and Cultivate: Other Important Considerations in Your Environment

- Chemicals in Daily Products
    - Detergent, Dish Soap, Makeup, and Hair Products: Replace these with clean, eco-friendly products. Look for those free from phthalates, parabens, and artificial fragrances, which are known to disrupt hormones.
    - Personal Care Products: Swap conventional brands for cleaner, natural options. Check labels for "paraben-free," "phthalate-free," and "fragrance-free" to minimize chemical exposure. Tampons need to be organic cotton and unscented. Makeup can also be a source of toxin exposure; read the labels.
- Water Quality
    - Good Options: Use a charcoal filter to remove basic contaminants from your water.
    - Best Option: Install a reverse osmosis filter for more thorough purification. Remember to add back in essential minerals and electrolytes, as these systems remove them along with contaminants.

- Staying Hydrated Safely: Encourage using glass or stainless steel water bottles to avoid plastic exposure.
- Air Quality
  - Air Filter: Use a high-quality HEPA air filter to remove dust, allergens, and VOCs from indoor air.
  - Air Duct Maintenance: Regularly clean or replace air ducts to reduce buildup of dust and allergens.
  - Radon Testing: If you live in an area with high radon levels, consider testing your home and installing a radon mitigation system if needed.

Radon is a gas that can be found in the basement of houses. So many people are not aware of this environmental toxin.

We just moved, and our new home turned up positive for radon in the basement. Just a little bit of radon in the environment can move throughout the entire house via the HVAC system and poison everyone in it. It needs to be mitigated by moving the air through to the outside. Get radon testing in your home.

- Sleep Environment
  - Phone and EMFs: Avoid sleeping with your phone next to your bed. Use airplane mode or keep it out of the room entirely to reduce EMF exposure. If you must have your phone on for emergencies, put it across the room.
  - Lights and Electronics: Keep your room dark and avoid lights from clocks or electronics. Use blackout curtains if necessary. Turn the Wi-Fi off at night. Wi-Fi exposure reduction hack: buy an inexpensive Christmas tree timer and connect it with your internet. Set the timer to turn the router off from 11:00 p.m. to 6:00 a.m. to reduce your exposure.

- Blue Light Reduction: Limit screen time before bed, or use blue light-blocking glasses to support melatonin production. Blue light prevents the pineal gland from releasing melatonin.
- Connecting with Safer Alternatives
  - Replacing Plastic with Glass: Choose glass storage containers, bottles, and cookware wherever possible to reduce exposure to hormone-disrupting chemicals found in plastics.
  - Choosing Cleaner Products: Switch to non-toxic cleaning and personal care products that don't contain endocrine disruptors. Include specific brands or certifications (like EWG Verified) that make choosing safer options easier.

Connecting with Your Circadian Rhythm to Optimize Hormones

Your body's internal clock, or circadian rhythm, is a 24-hour cycle that regulates various physiological processes, including hormone production. Syncing your daily habits with your circadian rhythm can have profound effects on your hormonal balance, energy levels, and overall well-being. Here's how you can connect with your circadian rhythm to optimize your hormones.

Think of your circadian rhythm as your body's conductor, guiding every instrument to play its part at the right time. Aligning with your natural rhythms—getting sunlight in the morning, avoiding blue light at night—is like keeping the conductor on stage. It ensures that your hormones, energy, and mood all follow the right cues, leading to a harmonious and vibrant performance.

How Your Circadian Rhythm Influences Hormones

Cortisol: Often called the "stress hormone," cortisol follows a natural circadian pattern. It peaks in the morning to wake you up and declines throughout the day to prepare you for sleep.

Melatonin: The "sleep hormone" rises in the evening when it gets dark, signaling to your body that it's time to wind down.

Insulin: The hormone that regulates blood sugar is more effective earlier in the day, making your body more efficient at processing food in the morning.

Estrogen, progesterone, and testosterone are influenced by your sleep-wake cycle, with optimal levels requiring consistent sleep and reduced stress. Disrupting your circadian rhythm through irregular sleep patterns, late-night screen time, or poor eating habits can throw off these hormone cycles, leading to fatigue, weight gain, mood swings, and more.

Steps to Sync Your Circadian Rhythm

Morning: Start Your Day with Natural Light

- Exposure to sunlight in the morning helps regulate cortisol levels and suppresses melatonin production, signaling to your brain that it's time to wake up.
- **Action Steps:**
  - Spend at least 10–15 minutes outside in the morning sunlight.
  - Open blinds or sit near a window if going outside isn't possible.

Midday: Align Meals with Insulin Sensitivity
- Your body processes carbohydrates more efficiently earlier in the day due to higher insulin sensitivity.
- **Action Steps:**
  - Make breakfast and lunch your largest meals, focusing on balanced macronutrients.
  - Avoid eating heavy meals late at night, as digestion slows down and can disrupt sleep.

Afternoon: Engage in Movement
- Moderate exercise during the morning or afternoon aligns with your body's peak physical performance and supports balanced cortisol levels.
- **Action Steps:**
  - Incorporate activities like walking or strength training into your afternoon routine.
  - Avoid high-intensity workouts late in the evening, as they may spike cortisol and disrupt sleep.

Evening: Limit Blue Light and Wind Down
- Exposure to artificial light, especially blue light from screens, suppresses melatonin production and delays your body's natural sleep cycle.
- **Action Steps:**
  - Use blue light-blocking glasses or switch devices to night mode after sunset.
  - Dim indoor lights and avoid screens at least one hour before bed.
  - Replace bright overhead lights with red or amber lighting in the evening.

Night: Create a Sleep Sanctuary
- Deep, restorative sleep is essential for hormone regulation, particularly for melatonin, growth hormone, and reproductive hormones.
- **Action Steps:**
  - Keep your bedroom dark, cool, and quiet.
  - Aim for seven to nine hours of quality sleep each night.
  - Establish a relaxing bedtime routine, such as reading, journaling, and prayer.

Practical Benefits of Circadian Rhythm Alignment

1. Balanced Cortisol: Reduced stress and improved focus during the day.
2. Better Sleep: Higher melatonin production leads to deeper, more restorative sleep.
3. Improved Metabolism: Enhanced insulin sensitivity supports stable blood sugar and weight management.
4. Reproductive Health: Hormones like estrogen and progesterone function optimally with consistent sleep-wake cycles.
5. Enhanced Mood and Energy: Reduced hormonal imbalances decrease fatigue and irritability.

Tips for Success

- Track your sleep and activity by using a wearable device or journal to monitor your sleep patterns and activity levels.
- Be consistent by waking up and going to bed at the same time every day, even on weekends.

Connecting with your circadian rhythm is one of the simplest, yet most effective, ways to optimize your hormones. By aligning your daily habits with your body's natural clock, you can enhance sleep, energy, and overall hormonal health. Remember that small changes, such as morning sunlight, balanced meals, and a consistent bedtime, can make a big difference in how you feel and function every day.

Just like the wok I finally threw away, little changes can make a big impact on our health. Letting go of the things we are used to or find convenient seems hard at first, but the more you put your health first, the more you will feel empowered.

Making healthier choices in your environment is like tending to a garden. Imagine each toxic product—like the nonstick wok or synthetic fragrances—as weeds. They may seem small, but left unchecked, they rob your garden of nutrients and vitality. Clearing out these weeds and replacing them with nurturing choices, like stainless steel cookware or natural cleaners, allows your health to flourish, just like healthy plants in rich, fertile soil.

Sometimes, letting go of conveniences like a favorite nonstick wok or your go-to fragrance feels like giving up part of your identity. But remember, Jesus invites us to give up burdens—not just spiritual burdens, but physical ones as well. Replacing toxic products with healthier options is an act of obedience, one that aligns your life with the abundant health and peace God desires for you.

Start with small changes. Swap out one thing at a time, whether it's your cookware, air fresheners, or sleep habits. As you begin to connect with better choices, you'll notice a transformation: not just in your environment, but in how you feel and thrive. Little by little, you're building a life that truly supports the vibrant health you were designed for.

And like the firefighters who reduced their toxic load through blood donation, it's never too late to act. Every step, no matter how small, helps. Toss the toxins and connect with a cleaner, healthier life. You are worth it, your health is worth it, and your body will thank you for every change you make.

Chapter Key Takeaways:

- Unburden your home: Replace toxic products for cleaner alternatives
- Smart changes like air filters or natural cleaners to make a difference
- Optimize your hormones: Sync healthy habits with your circadian rhythm

CHAPTER 3

Cultivate a Healthy Habitat

In peace I will lie down and sleep, for you alone,
LORD, make me dwell in safety.

—Psalm 4:8 (NIV)

Any other health care night shift workers out there? When I started having more and more kids, night shift became the most convenient option as a working mother. It also gave me the flexibility to make it to all their activities and get them ready for school. Did you know that night shift has actually been found to be a carcinogen? Working night shift is not cultivating a healthy environment or promoting healthy hormones.

What else in our environment can cause harm to our hormones?

And he shall examine the disease.
And if the disease is in the walls of the house with greenish or reddish spots, and if it appears to be deeper than the surface, then the priest shall go out of the house to the door of the house and shut up the house seven days.

—Leviticus 14:37 (CSB)

Cultivate a Mold-Free Environment

Mold is a prevalent issue in U.S. homes. According to the National Institute for Occupational Safety and Health (NIOSH), approximately 47% of residential buildings in the United States exhibit signs of dampness or mold. This statistic underscores the widespread nature of mold problems across the country.

When I was practicing full time in northwest Ohio, which used to be a swamp, mold was a huge issue. It was frustrating for all involved, as remediation can be difficult and expensive. A lot of people were in denial about it.

I grew up in a beautiful house that, sadly, grew mold. We didn't have air-conditioning or good venting in my bathroom. My bathroom had mushrooms growing in the corner and carpet! It doesn't matter when your house was built or how beautiful it is; it could still have mold, which can poison your body and negatively affect your hormones.

What Are Mycotoxins?

Mycotoxins are toxic chemicals produced by certain molds that grow in damp conditions or on improperly stored foods. Think of them as the "chemical defense weapons" molds use to outcompete other microorganisms. When you're exposed to mold or its toxins—through inhalation, skin contact, or food—it's like introducing unwanted players into your body's hormonal orchestra.

Zearalenone (ZEN) is a toxin—a mycotoxin produced by *Fusarium* molds that grow on grains like corn and wheat. It acts as a *xenoestrogen* (foreign estrogen), which means it can mimic estrogen in the body. Here's what happens.

Estrogen Mimicry: Imagine estrogen as the correct key for a lock (the estrogen receptor). Zearalenone is a counterfeit key. It fits into the receptor, but it doesn't open the door in the normal way. Instead, it disrupts the usual signaling.

If you're in perimenopause and already experiencing fluctuating estrogen levels, Zearalenone can act like an unruly locksmith, confusing your body's hormonal balance even more. This false estrogen signal is the "disruptor" of hormones, which can worsen symptoms.

Symptoms of Estrogen Dominance

This mimicry can lead to estrogen dominance symptoms, even when your actual estrogen levels are low, exacerbating issues like mood swings, irregular periods, breast tenderness, and hot flashes—all common during perimenopause.

Gut Health and Mycotoxins

Your gut is a carefully balanced ecosystem, with microbes acting as the gatekeepers of health. Mycotoxins can upset this balance in several ways:

- Mycotoxins damage the gut lining, similar to how a storm breaks down the walls of a dam. This allows toxins, partially digested food, and inflammatory molecules to leak into the bloodstream, creating systemic inflammation.
- Zearalenone and other mycotoxins reduce beneficial bacteria, such as *Lactobacillus* and *Bifidobacterium*, while allowing harmful bacteria and yeasts like *Candida* to thrive. This microbial imbalance can worsen hormone regulation since gut bacteria help metabolize and regulate estrogen levels through the estrobolome (gut bacteria that manage the amount of estrogen that exits and remains in your body).

The "musty smell" associated with mold is due to volatile organic compounds (VOCs). These are small, airborne chemicals that molds release as part of their metabolic processes.

- VOCs serve as a "smoke signal" indicating that mold is actively producing toxins in the environment.

- When you inhale VOCs, they can enter your bloodstream through your lungs and disrupt systems, especially in sensitive individuals. Symptoms can include headaches, fatigue, and respiratory issues, which may indirectly affect hormone balance.

How Mold Affects Hormones

Perimenopause is already a time of hormonal flux, with the body transitioning from regular menstrual cycles to menopause. Mycotoxins can amplify the chaos:

- Mycotoxins stress the hypothalamic-pituitary-adrenal (HPA) axis—the body's stress response system that links the brain to the adrenal glands. The HPA axis regulates cortisol. Elevated cortisol (chronic stress) further dysregulates the HPA axis, particularly estrogen, progesterone, and testosterone levels. This dysfunction can intensify perimenopausal symptoms (fatigue, anxiety, sleep disturbance, high cortisol), making hormonal stability difficult.
- Mycotoxins burden the liver, which is responsible for breaking down and eliminating excess estrogen. If the liver is overwhelmed, estrogen clearance slows, leading to estrogen dominance.

Hormone Effects of Mycotoxins

Zearalenone binds with estrogen receptors, but its effects can vary:

- ERα vs. ERβ: These are two types of estrogen receptors.
  - ERα (alpha): Promotes cell growth and proliferation, especially in breast and uterine tissue.
  - ERβ (beta): Acts as a regulator or "brake" on growth.
  - Zearalenone preferentially activates ERα, which may lead to estrogen-like effects such as increased cell growth or a heightened risk of hormone-sensitive conditions like fibroids or endometriosis.

Can zearalenone feminize men? Yes, zearalenone can mimic estrogen's effects and cause physiological feminization in males under certain conditions:

- Excess estrogenic signaling can stimulate breast tissue growth, called gynecomastia.
- Overactive estrogen signaling can suppress testosterone production, leading to changes in muscle mass, libido, and secondary sexual characteristics.
- Zearalenone exposure in high doses has been linked to infertility and reduced sperm quality in animal studies.

Recap: Beware of Mold and How You Can Protect Your Health

- Avoid Moldy Environments: The musty smell signals active mold growth and VOC release. Ensure proper ventilation and address water damage promptly, not only in your home but also at work and school.
- Gut Support: Probiotics, prebiotics, and fermented foods can help restore microbiome balance, and address gut dysbiosis. Peptides like BPC157, KPV, and larazotide can help support gut health.
- Liver Support: Enhance detoxification pathways with cruciferous vegetables (broccoli, kale) and antioxidants (e.g., glutathione).
- Binders for Mycotoxins: Activated charcoal, bentonite clay, and chlorella may help reduce toxin absorption in the gut. Check out my resources for my gut protocol.

Preventing Mold in Your Home

Keep mold away by controlling moisture, ensuring ventilation, and maintaining your home properly.

1. Control Humidity: Keep indoor humidity between 30% and 50%, use dehumidifiers, and ventilate kitchens, bathrooms, and laundry rooms.
2. Fix Leaks and Dry Spills Quickly: Repair leaks immediately and dry wet surfaces within 24 hours.
3. Improve Air Circulation: Open windows, use fans, and keep HVAC vents unblocked.
4. Waterproof Problem Areas: Seal basements, ensure that landscaping slopes away from the house, and install sump pumps.
5. Prevent Condensation: Insulate pipes, seal windows, and use vapor barriers.
6. Maintain HVAC Systems: Replace filters every one to three months, service units annually, and use HEPA filters.
7. Avoid Carpeting in Damp Areas: Use mold-resistant flooring and dry wet carpets immediately.
8. Monitor Moisture-Prone Areas: Clean bathrooms with mold-killing products and remove moisture-trapping clutter.
9. Use Mold-Resistant Materials: Apply mold-resistant paint, drywall, and insulation.
10. Inspect and Maintain Property Regularly: Check for musty odors, discoloration, and water damage, and perform seasonal maintenance.

Daisy was struggling during perimenopause. Her health had started declining a few years ago, and she didn't know why. She had headaches, fatigue, and problems with her cycle. When she came to me, she had tried everything she could over the counter and from reading online. She was barely able to walk into my office. After taking an integrative medical history, I was concerned about mold and had her test for mycotoxins and mold in her home.

Mold was found in the master bedroom closet. She and her husband were being affected the most, but, unfortunately, the kids were also struggling. The mold she was dealing with produced zearalenone, which was affecting her hormones. The key to getting her to even be able to function was to start progesterone during the luteal phase. She was able to function enough to start the detox process and heal from the mold. Daisy's hormones were able to self-regulate again. She is now thriving in a remediated house and knows to be on the lookout for mold.

Cultivate a Sweet Sleep Environment

Ada came to me very anxious during perimenopause. She would go to bed late and wake up at 4:00 a.m. to get her workout in. She had done this for years, so she didn't connect the dots that it might be causing a problem. We discussed her sleep schedule and worked on adjusting it so that she was getting eight hours each night. Once her sleep was more balanced, her anxiety improved.

Sleep is essential during perimenopause and for longevity, as it directly impacts hormonal balance, metabolic health, cognitive function, and overall well-being.

During perimenopause, fluctuations in estrogen and progesterone can disrupt sleep patterns, leading to insomnia, night sweats, and increased cortisol levels, which accelerate aging and inflammation.

Poor sleep quality contributes to weight gain, insulin resistance, and increased cardiovascular risk, all of which are concerns during this transition.

Deep sleep is crucial for cellular repair, immune function, and reducing oxidative stress, which are key factors in healthy aging and longevity.

Additionally, REM sleep supports memory consolidation and emotional regulation, reducing the risk of neurodegenerative diseases like Alzheimer's.

Prioritizing quality sleep can help stabilize hormones, support metabolism, and promote resilience against age-related decline, making it a cornerstone of healthy aging and optimal well-being.

Here's an easy way to remember the optimal sleep distribution and how each stage works in an eight-hour sleep:

"2-4-2 Rule for 8 Hours"
- 2 Hours REM: *Brain Boost*
- 4 Hours Light (NREM Stage 2): *Refresh & Recharge*
- 2 Hours Deep (NREM Stage 3): *Body Repair*

When someone is at the gym and they are walking around the track, just because they are at the gym doesn't mean they are getting good exercise. In a similar way, you can be in bed "sleeping," but not getting restorative sleep. This is why a sleep tracker can be helpful.

Sleep Explained

NREM Sleep (75% of the Night)

As we start to fall asleep, we enter Non-Rapid Eye Movement (NREM) sleep, which makes up the first three stages and accounts for 75% of our sleep. This phase is crucial for physical restoration.

- Stages:
  - Stage 1: Light sleep, where we begin to drift off. Eye movement and muscle activity slow.
  - Stage 2: A deeper phase, where breathing and heart rate continue to slow, and the body begins to relax more.
  - Stage 3 (Deep Sleep): The deepest sleep stage, where the body focuses on physical repair and immune support.
- Hormones Released: During NREM, growth hormone is released, which is essential for growth, muscle repair, and overall development.

- Benefits: NREM sleep is essential for physical recovery, tissue repair, and immune function. It helps prepare the body for the next day's activities.

REM Sleep (25% of the Night)

- Overview: REM sleep, or Rapid Eye Movement sleep, typically begins 90 minutes after falling asleep. REM phases recur about every 90 minutes throughout the night, each cycle getting longer as the night progresses.
- Key Characteristics:
    - Brain Activity: The brain is highly active, similar to wakefulness, which is why dreaming occurs during REM sleep.
    - Eye Movement: The eyes dart back and forth rapidly under the eyelids.
    - Body Relaxation: The body becomes immobile, as muscles are "turned off" to prevent movement during dreams.
- Benefits: REM sleep restores energy to the brain and body, supporting learning, memory consolidation, and emotional regulation. It's also critical for next-day performance, aiding cognitive function, problem-solving, and overall mood balance.

Quick Recap:

- NREM Sleep: 75% of the night. Physical repair and growth happens through hormone release, divided into stages 1–3.
- REM Sleep: 25% of the night. Mental and emotional recovery happens in this stage where the brain is active, dreams occur, and the body is immobile.

Steps to Improve Sleep

1. Create a Sleep Sanctuary: Focus on creating a sleep-friendly environment by using calming colors, limiting artificial light, and reducing noise. Incorporate natural fabrics for bedding and consider air-purifying plants.

2. Sleep Routine: Discuss the importance of a consistent sleep schedule, winding down an hour before bed, and reducing EMF exposure for better quality sleep.
3. Track Your Progress: Use a sleep journal and a sleep tracker to observe how changes in your sleep environment impact sleep quality, noting improvements in energy, mood, and focus.
4. Use Red Lights at Night: Blue light from screens and bright white lights can disrupt melatonin production, making it harder to fall asleep. Switching to red bulbs in the evening helps minimize blue light exposure, signaling to your body that it's time to wind down.

He told them still another parable: "The kingdom of heaven is like yeast that a woman took and mixed into about sixty pounds of flour until it worked all through the dough.

—Matthew 13:33 (NIV)

Cultivating this new nontoxic lifestyle can seem challenging. But if you change one thing, it will work into your everyday activities, like the yeast mixing into the wheat in the parable. Before you know it, you will be inspiring others.

It was amazing to watch Catherine blossom while working with her. She slowly switched her products over time. First, she threw away the air fresheners in her car. Then, she bought an air filter for her home. She also changed her Tupperware to glassware.

While she was changing her environment, she was focusing on sleep. She had usually been waking up in the middle of the night to pee, but once we got her blood sugar and hormones balanced, she was finally sleeping all night. She even lost 15 pounds as a bonus! Her family also started making switches, and before you knew it, they all even went gluten-free with her. She was committed to making the changes, and her persistence paid off. Catherine's health was a priority now.

Smart Sleep Supplementation

Supplements can be a great support for improving sleep, especially at the beginning of your healing journey. While they're not a replacement for addressing poor sleep habits or lifestyle factors, they can help get your body back into a healthy rhythm. Here are a few of my go-to options:

L-theanine

- An amino acid commonly found in teas
- Has anxiolytic (anxiety-reducing) effects via the induction of α brain waves without the additives and other side effects associated with conventional sleep inducers
- No daytime drowsiness
- Promotes good quality of sleep through anxiolysis, not sedation
- Dosing: 100–200 mg nightly

DHH-B (Dihydrohonokiol-B)

- DHH-B boosts the activity of gamma-aminobutyric acid (GABA), a crucial inhibitory neurotransmitter that helps calm neuronal excitability. By enhancing GABA function, DHH-B supports better sleep quality and helps reduce anxiety levels.
- Dosing: 15 mg before bedtime.

Passionflower extract

- Used for sleep and anxiety
- Non-sedating
- Activates GABA receptors and promotes positive effects on circadian rhythms
- Usually combined with lemon balm and valerian for sleep
- Passionflower is gentle for children also
- Dosing: 500 mg capsule at bedtime or 1 cup of tea before bed

Magnesium

- Can improve sleep quality
- Maintains healthy levels of GABA
- Also helps with depression and anxiety
- Most people are magnesium deficient
- Dosing: 200–400 mg in the evening

Melatonin

- A hormone made in the pineal gland
- Has antioxidant, immune, and anti-inflammatory properties
- Is correlated with the sleep-wake cycle; synchronizes the body's internal clock
- Dosing: 1–10 mg thirty minutes prior to bed

Progesterone

- Progesterone is converted into allopregnanolone in the brain.
- Allopregnanolone is a neuroactive steroid that has a high affinity for GABA receptors, which are responsible for promoting calmness and relaxation.
- By acting on GABA receptors, allopregnanolone helps lower stress responses, enhance mood stability, and promote deeper, more restful sleep, including better REM continuity.
- Dosing: 75–200 mg E4M capsules (depends on hormone levels, pre- or post-menopausal: test first!)

Lavender essential oil

- Can help with sleep and anxiety
- Use topically in a carrier oil or in a diffuser

Your environment has a profound impact on your hormones—and, ultimately, your health and peace of mind. From hidden mold to disrupted sleep, what surrounds you shapes what's happening inside you. But healing begins with awareness and small, intentional steps. Whether it's tossing out fragrance-laden products, investing in better sleep hygiene, or cleaning up hidden toxins, these decisions add up.

God calls us to live with wisdom and discernment, not fear. Like yeast working its way through dough, even one change—done in faith—can multiply into a complete transformation. Your body was designed by a God who heals, and each night of restorative sleep, each detoxified corner of your home, is a step back into alignment with that design.

Chapter Key Takeaways:

- Beware of mycotoxins (made by mold) as they can intensify hormone imbalance
- Be proactive and prevent mold from taking hold in your home.
- Support the quality of your sleep via habits and supplement use

PART 2:
BODY

So, whether you eat or drink, or whatever you do, do all to the glory of God.

—1 Corinthians 10:31 (NIV)

What we put in our body can create inflammation, or it can help heal inflammation. It's very important that we treat our body that God created with respect and honor as precious. Whatever we are eating or drinking, we should glorify Him.

Julie came to me with her hormones a mess. She was having very short cycles of 21 days. Worse yet, she was getting very irritable during the last week before her period. She also had bad constipation and belly bloat. She was hesitant to change her diet, but I assured her that a new focus on liver health and gut health would help her hormones balance out. As a result of my advice, she went 100% gluten free, focusing on healthy fats and protein. After three months, she extended her cycle back to 28 days and felt less inflamed. No more belly bloat either!

THE HORMONAL FARM: A WELL-BALANCED ECOSYSTEM

Imagine your body as a large, diverse farm, with each hormone acting as a key player in keeping the farm running smoothly. Just like a farm requires a balance of resources and careful management, the body relies on its hormones to work together, creating a productive, healthy environment.

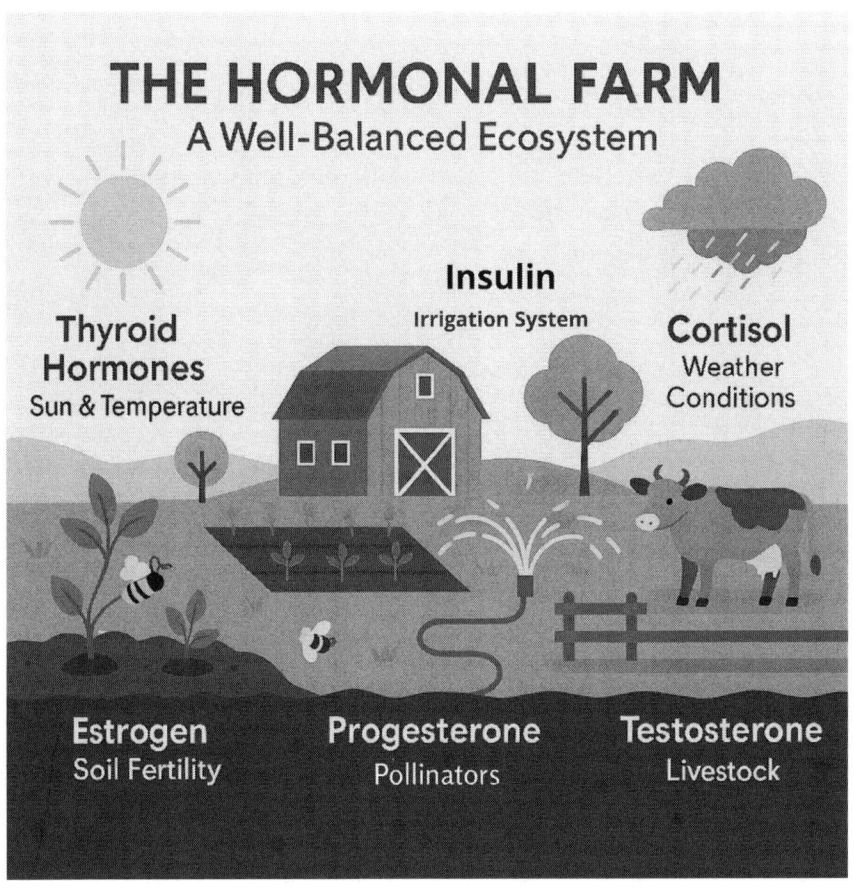

Key Roles on the Hormonal Farm:

- Thyroid Hormones (Sunlight and Temperature): The thyroid acts like the sun and temperature on the farm, setting the pace for growth and activity. Just as plants need the right amount of sunlight and warmth to grow properly, the body depends on thyroid hormones to regulate metabolism, energy, and temperature. Too much "sunlight" (hyperthyroidism) can burn out the plants, while too little (hypothyroidism) slows everything down, making the farm sluggish.

- Insulin (Irrigation System): Insulin works like the irrigation system, delivering water (glucose) to all parts of the farm. It helps ensure that each crop and animal has the energy to grow and thrive. If the irrigation system malfunctions, either by providing too much water (high insulin) or not enough (insulin resistance), parts of the farm might become overgrown, dry up, or wilt, disrupting the farm's balance.
- Sex Hormones (Fertile Soil and Pollinators):
    - Estrogen (Soil Fertility): Estrogen is like the fertile soil, rich in nutrients and necessary for the health of many plants and animals. It supports growth, reproduction, and resilience across the farm. Without healthy, fertile soil, plants may struggle to grow, and animals may lack the nutrients they need, causing an imbalance in the farm ecosystem.
    - Progesterone (Pollinators): Progesterone acts like bees and other pollinators, helping ensure that the crops are productive and supporting balance in the reproductive cycle. If the pollinators don't visit (low progesterone), crops may not fully ripen, leading to irregular growth patterns and affecting the farm's output.
    - Testosterone (Livestock): Testosterone acts like the livestock on the farm, providing power, strength, and productivity. The animals bring vitality to the farm, supporting its daily tasks and helping it thrive. If there's an imbalance (too few or too many animals), the farm's productivity and energy levels can be affected, impacting everything from growth to reproduction.
- Cortisol (Weather Conditions): Cortisol functions like the weather on the farm, responding to stress and changes. When storms (stress) hit, cortisol rises to help the farm manage the impact, providing resilience. But if the "storm" lasts too long (chronic stress), it can erode the soil, damage crops, and overwork the animals, throwing the entire ecosystem out of balance.

CHAPTER 4
Cleanse from Within

Do you not know that your bodies are temples of the Holy Spirit, who is in you, whom you have received from God? You are not your own; you were bought at a price. Therefore, honor God with your bodies.

1 Corinthians 6:19–20 (NIV)

Just as a farm manager oversees all aspects of the farm's operation, integrative medicine helps maintain the health of this complex hormonal ecosystem. Through nutrition (fertilizers), supplements (supportive tools), and lifestyle practices (farm management techniques), we can support each hormone's role. This careful management ensures that the farm remains balanced, productive, and ready to adapt to challenges.

One of my patients, Susan, did not want to give up gluten. She would come back to appointments almost gluten free, but cheat on the weekends, eating gluten and not staying committed to her health. "It doesn't affect me. I don't think it's a big deal," she would say. However, as we will learn in this chapter, a little bit of gluten, is like a little bit of poison to the gut and can wreak havoc!

Scripture reminds us that we are stewards of our bodies—temples of the Holy Spirit. In a world filled with toxins and processed food, it's essential that we remain informed and intentional.

Many of us have unknowingly turned food into an idol, living to eat instead of eating to live. While God designed food to be a gift—something to nourish us and even bring joy through fellowship—it's easy to cross the line into excess or dependence.

I personally think GMOs, seed oils, food dyes, and modern-day gluten are part of the enemy's plan to destroy our physical body, making us tired and weary.

According to the Environmental Working Group, food lobbyists spent $101 million in 2015 to oppose labeling of GMO foods. There is big money in making us sick. The good news? Knowledge is power!

What Are GMO Crops?

According to USDA.gov as of this writing, "By 2020 (the most recent year for which data are available), about 55 percent of the total harvested cropland in the United States was grown with varieties having at least one GM (genetically modified) trait. The most prevalent GM traits are herbicide tolerance and insect resistance."

Herbicide tolerance and insect resistance mean that farmers can spray as much pesticide as they want on the crops. This means more glyphosate (Roundup) in our waterways and in the rain. Private seed companies drive this trend, since seed prices for GM crops are very expensive.

I often think back to the "good old days" of middle school—when life felt simpler, and our food wasn't packed with additives, dyes, and chemicals. I remind my patients that food today isn't what it used to be. Not only is much of it toxic, but it's also void of essential micronutrients due to over farming and soil that's been depleted of life. Our environment and food system have changed—and our health is paying the price.

GMOs erupted in the U.S. in 1996 with corn, soybeans, and cotton. Since then, more have been added.

USDA Organic and Non-GMO Label Meanings

What Does USDA Organic and Non-GMO Mean on the Label?

A. USDA Organic
1. This label signifies that a product is certified to meet strict organic farming and production standards set by the U.S. Department of Agriculture (USDA).
2. Key Criteria:
   i. No synthetic fertilizers, pesticides, or herbicides used.
   ii. No genetically modified organisms (GMOs) allowed.
   iii. Animals are raised in conditions that allow natural behaviors, with organic feed and no anitbiotics or hormones.
   iv. No artificial preservatives, colors, or flavors in processed products.

B. Non-GMO
1. This label means the product does not contain genetically modified organisms.
2. It focuses solely on the absence of GMOs and does not consider broader farming practices such as pesticide use or animal welfare, which are covered by organic certification.

C. What is Greenwashing? By definition greenwashing is a marketing tactic where companies make misleading or exaggerated claims about how environmentally friendly their products, services, or practices are to appeal to eco-conscious consumers.

D. Common Examples
   1. Using vague terms like "natural" or "eco-friendly" without certification.
   2. Displaying green colors, leaves, or other eco-themed designs on packaging to suggest sustainability.
   3. Highlighting one environmentally friendly aspect while ignoring significant environmental harm elsewhere in the production process.

E. Why It Matters: Greenwashing can mislead consumers into thinking they're making environmentally responsible choices when the claims lack substance or verification. Always look for credible certifications like USDA Organic, Non-GMO Project Verified, or Fair Trade for assurance.

Glyphosate

Imagine your gut lining as a strong yet delicate screen door. This screen is designed to let in fresh air (nutrients) and keep out bugs (toxins and harmful microbes). Glyphosate, a widely used herbicide and the active ingredient in Roundup, acts like a mischievous kid poking holes in this screen. The result? Toxins, undigested food particles, and harmful bacteria can sneak through, triggering a cascade of health problems often referred to as *leaky gut*.

As if perimenopause wasn't challenging enough, the presence of glyphosate in our food and environment may exacerbate the hormonal imbalances that come with this transitional phase. During perimenopause, the body experiences fluctuating levels of estrogen, progesterone, and other hormones, making women more susceptible to external influences like endocrine disruptors.

Glyphosate, originally designed as an herbicide, has also been implicated in hormone disruption. Here's how this chemical may impact hormones and intensify perimenopausal symptoms.

Glyphosate as an Endocrine Disruptor

Endocrine disruptors are chemicals that interfere with the body's hormone production, signaling, or metabolism. Glyphosate has been shown to mimic and disrupt hormonal pathways, particularly those involving estrogen.

Glyphosate can act as a xenoestrogen—a synthetic compound that mimics estrogen. By binding to estrogen receptors, it may cause overstimulation or block natural estrogen's effects. This interference can exacerbate common perimenopausal symptoms such as:

- Mood swings and anxiety
- Hot flashes and night sweats
- Irregular periods and heavier bleeding

Perimenopause often brings changes in thyroid function, which controls metabolism, energy levels, and mood. Glyphosate may further burden the thyroid by chelating iodine, a mineral essential for thyroid hormone production, and inducing oxidative stress, which can damage thyroid cells.

During perimenopause, the adrenal glands take on a greater role in producing sex hormones as ovarian function declines. Glyphosate exposure has been linked to adrenal stress and reduced production of key hormones like cortisol and DHEA (a precursor to estrogen and testosterone) leading to worsening perimenopausal fatigue, weight gain, and low libido.

The Gut-Hormone Axis in Perimenopause

The gut and hormones are deeply interconnected, forming what is known as the gut-hormone axis. Damage to the gut lining and microbiome caused by glyphosate can have a domino effect on hormone health leading to estrobolome disruption, impaired nutrient absorption, and increased inflammation.

The estrobolome refers to the gut bacteria responsible for metabolizing and regulating estrogen. Glyphosate-induced dysbiosis can disrupt this process, leading to:

- Estrogen dominance (high estrogen relative to progesterone), which is linked to heavy periods, bloating, and breast tenderness
- Difficulty detoxifying estrogen, exacerbating hormone-related symptoms

Glyphosate chelates minerals like zinc and magnesium, which are critical for hormone production and regulation. These deficiencies can worsen:

- Hot flashes (linked to magnesium deficiency)
- Mood swings and irritability (associated with low zinc levels)

Chronic inflammation caused by leaky gut and dysbiosis may further disrupt hormone signaling and increase the risk of conditions like endometriosis or fibroids.

Wheat, as a major source of glyphosate exposure due to pre-harvest spraying, poses a unique risk to hormonal health during perimenopause. High glyphosate residues in wheat-based products can contribute to leaky gut and amplify estrogen imbalances. Women in perimenopause may benefit significantly from a gluten-free diet, as it can:

- Reduce glyphosate exposure, giving the gut a chance to heal
- Stabilize blood sugar levels, which is critical for balancing hormones
- Lower systemic inflammation, improving symptoms like bloating, joint pain, and fatigue

Practical Steps for Reducing Glyphosate's Impact During Perimenopause

1. Adopt an Organic Diet: Organic foods are free from glyphosate residues and other endocrine-disrupting pesticides. Check the labels for oats and make sure they are organic, or you will be getting a dose of glyphosate with your oats!
2. Go Gluten-Free: Eliminating wheat and gluten-containing grains can reduce glyphosate exposure and support gut health.

Why Gluten Can Lead to Intestinal Permeability

Gliadin and Zonulin Release:

Gluten contains a protein called gliadin. In susceptible individuals, gliadin interacts with the intestinal lining and triggers the release of zonulin, a protein that regulates the tight junctions (gatekeepers) between intestinal cells.

Tight Junction Disruption:

Zonulin loosens these tight junctions, leading to increased intestinal permeability (a.k.a. leaky gut).

A leaky gut allows substances like partially digested food or bacterial toxins to enter the bloodstream, which can provoke inflammation and immune responses.

How to Support Your Gut:
1. Include Detox Pathways: Incorporate foods and supplements that aid in hormone detoxification, such as:
    - Cruciferous vegetables (e.g., broccoli, cauliflower) for estrogen metabolism.
    - Magnesium and zinc supplements to support adrenal and thyroid health.
2. Take probiotics to restore the estrobolome.

3. Strengthen Gut Health: Use gut-healing protocols, including bone broth, collagen, and L-glutamine, to repair the intestinal lining.
    - Minimize Processed Foods: These often contain higher levels of glyphosate residues and fewer nutrients.

Non-Celiac Gluten Sensitivity (NCGS) vs. Celiac Disease

Celiac Disease (CD):

- An autoimmune disorder where gluten (a protein in wheat, barley, and rye) triggers an immune response that damages the lining of the small intestine.
- Leads to nutrient malabsorption, diarrhea, bloating, and systemic issues like fatigue or anemia.
- Diagnosed via blood tests (antibodies like tTG-IgA) and intestinal biopsy, showing villous atrophy.

Non-Celiac Gluten Sensitivity (NCGS):

- A condition where people experience symptoms similar to CD (e.g., bloating, fatigue, abdominal pain) but without the autoimmune response or intestinal damage seen in CD.
- The exact mechanism is unclear, but it may involve innate immune activation or non-gluten components in wheat. It may also have something to do with glyphosate.

Why am I spending so much time talking about the dangers of glyphosate and the health concerns of gluten? Because I want you to eliminate gluten from your diet. When we get into cycle syncing, I will give you a specific diet plan to help you balance your hormones. When you cut out gluten, you also cut out a lot of carbohydrates. Replacing carbs with healthy fats and protein will help keep your blood sugar balanced.

Gut health is so important for balancing hormones. So, what do I recommend for your diet? It depends.

For someone who has Hashimoto's thyroiditis, I would recommend eliminating gluten forever, as the body can get confused sometimes with gluten!

For some other people, once their gut is truly healed, they may be able to add sourdough or ancient grains back in. However, it is crucial to make sure they are not sprayed with pesticides, or else the cycle will start again.

For everyone, avoiding processed foods and the ingredients I mentioned previously will help. I find that my patients do best when they follow a whole foods diet and make sure to focus on the correct vegetables, healthy fats, and protein.

I have included some plans and macros in this book. The macros do matter. I think it's wild when people say that it's calories in, calories out. This is not what we see in practice. Drinking 100 calories of soda with high fructose corn syrup does not equal 100 calories of a ribeye. One will cause inflammation in the body, while the other is giving your body building blocks of amino acids to make neurotransmitters, provide B vitamins, and keep you satisfied.

Easy Swaps for Going Gluten Free

FOOD	REGULAR GLUTEN-FREE SWAP	LOWER-CARB ALTERNATIVE	ANIMAL-BASED OR CARNIVORE OPTION
PIZZA	Gluten-free crust (rice flour, tapioca, or oat-based)	Low-carb crust (cauliflower, almond flour, or cheese-based crust)	Meat crust (e.g., ground chicken, beef, or pork formed into a crust)
MAC AND CHEESE	Gluten-free pasta (chickpea, lentil, or corn-based)	Zucchini noodles, spaghetti squash, or shirataki noodles with cheese sauce	Meat "pasta" (ground beef or shredded chicken topped with cheese)
BREAD	Gluten-free bread (made with rice or tapioca flour)	Low-carb bread (almond flour, coconut flour, or protein bread)	Cloud bread (made with eggs and cream cheese)
CRACKERS	Gluten-free crackers (seed or rice-based)	Low-carb crackers (cheese crisps, flaxseed crackers)	Cheese crisps (baked slices of cheese)
PASTA	Gluten-free pasta (quinoa, corn, or rice-based)	Zoodles (zucchini noodles), spaghetti squash, or shirataki noodles	Ground meat or organ meats layered like lasagna
TORTILLAS/WRAPS	Gluten-free tortillas (corn or cassava-based)	Low-carb tortillas (coconut flour, almond flour, or egg wraps)	Egg wraps or deli meat slices
CEREAL	Gluten-free cereal (made from rice or corn)	Low-carb granola (made from nuts and seeds)	Pork rinds with whole milk
PANCAKES	Gluten-free pancakes (made with rice or oat flour)	Low-carb pancakes (almond flour or coconut flour-based)	Egg-based pancakes (eggs with cream cheese or ricotta)

FOOD	REGULAR GLUTEN-FREE SWAP	LOWER-CARB ALTERNATIVE	ANIMAL-BASED OR CARNIVORE OPTION
SNACKS	Gluten-free snacks (rice crackers, popcorn)	Low-carb snacks (nuts, seeds, veggie chips, or olives)	Beef jerky, pork rinds, or hard-boiled eggs
COOKIES	Gluten-free cookies (rice flour, oat-based)	Low-carb cookies (almond flour, coconut flour, or seed-based)	No-sugar-added cheese crisps with a sweetener like stevia if needed
DESSERTS	Gluten-free desserts (fruit-based pies, rice flour cakes)	Low-carb desserts (keto cakes, cheesecake with almond flour crusts)	Whipped cream, egg-based soufflés
BURGERS	Gluten-free buns (rice or potato flour-based)	Lettuce wraps or low-carb buns (made from almond or coconut flour)	Burger patties without buns

*use organic ingredients, including grass fed/finished meat without nitrites

Time to Cleanse, Connect, and Cultivate with Liver Detoxification

It is important for your liver to be operating properly. As we discussed earlier, environmental toxins like parabens and mycotoxins gunk up your liver. Sometimes your body just needs a chance to detox.

Emily came to me tired, and her hormones were off. I got her started on a liver cleanse. She lost 11 pounds due to inflammation and got her energy back. Over time, I've seen repeatedly that when the liver becomes sluggish or overburdened—from toxins, poor diet, or hormonal imbalances—your body can hold on to excess weight, inflammation, and fat. By supporting healthy liver detoxification pathways, you can improve hormone metabolism, reduce inflammatory load, and make it easier for your body to release stored weight and regain vitality.

ESTROGEN DETOXIFICATION: THE HORMONAL WASTE MANAGEMENT SYSTEM

Think of your body as a bustling city. In this example, estrogen is an essential product manufactured in factories (your ovaries, adrenal glands, and fat tissues). Just like any product, there are leftovers and packaging that need to be managed once estrogen has done its job. If this waste isn't properly collected, sorted, processed, and discarded, it can accumulate and create chaos in the city (your body).

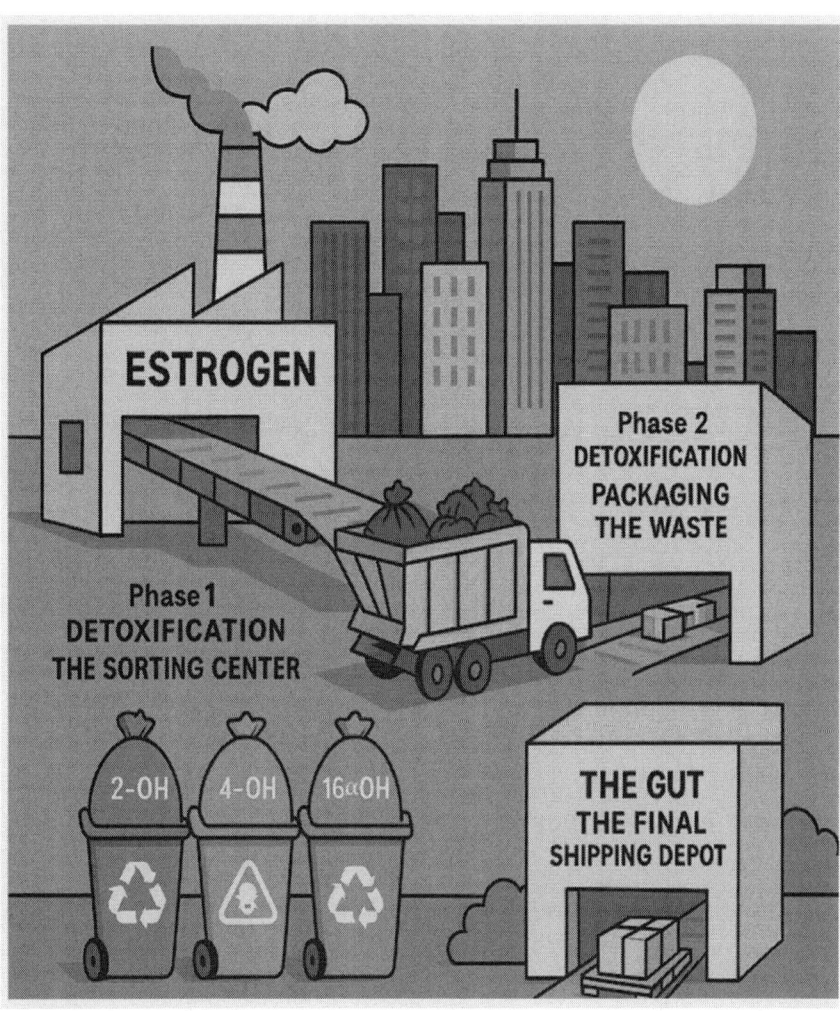

Phase 1 Detoxification: The Sorting Center

What Happens: In the liver, enzymes from the cytochrome P450 family perform the first step of estrogen detox. This is like a factory where waste products are "tagged" or "broken down" into smaller, easier-to-handle forms. However, these intermediate products can be unstable, like a half-filled garbage bag that might spill if not quickly handled.

The Three Estrogen "Trash Bins"

1. 2-OH (2-Hydroxyestrone): The "green" bin (recyclable). This is the safest form, promoting hormonal balance and minimal damage.
2. 4-OH (4-Hydroxyestrone): The "hazardous waste" bin. It can leak into the system and cause harm, including DNA damage, if not quickly processed and removed.
3. 16α-OH (16-alpha-Hydroxyestrone): The "bulky trash" bin. This form is less harmful but can still lead to issues like excessive tissue growth (e.g., fibroids or cancer risk).

If Phase 1 is sluggish or overly active, you may end up with an overflow of harmful intermediates. This is why antioxidants are critical—they act like safety officers, preventing these intermediates from causing oxidative damage.

Think of the metabolites like this: 2-OH (the good), 16α-OH (the bad), and 4-OH (the ugly). You want to go down mostly the good pathway. Estrogen metabolite testing is a window into your personalized estrogen detoxification pathways.

Phase 2 Detoxification: Packaging the Waste

What Happens: Now that the "garbage" is sorted, it's time to package it for transport. The liver uses enzymes that "wrap up" the estrogen metabolites with chemical groups such as:

- Methylation: Adds a "methyl tag" for safe shipping.
- Glucuronidation: Like bubble wrap, it secures the metabolites in a water-soluble form.
- Sulfation: Adds a sulfur tag, acting as a biohazard sticker.

Imagine the liver as a packaging plant with conveyor belts:

1. Estrogen intermediates come in from Phase 1.
2. The enzymes (workers) package each item based on its type.
3. They're loaded onto trucks (bile or bloodstream) for transport out of the body.

If Phase 2 is inefficient, the hazardous estrogen intermediates remain unpackaged, roaming the system and causing havoc. These "unfinished" estrogen byproducts can damage cells, increase inflammation, and contribute to hormone-related problems like PMS, weight gain, and even higher cancer risk over time. Nutrients like B vitamins (especially B6, B12, and folate), magnesium, and SAMe are critical because they fuel the enzymes that finish processing and safely package estrogen for elimination.

The Gut: The Final Shipping Depot

Packaged estrogen metabolites arrive at the gut via bile (a digestive juice produced by the liver). Here, the gut microbiome acts like customs officers, ensuring that the "garbage" is shipped out of the body in the stool.

The Role of Beta-Glucuronidase

Sometimes, mischievous bacteria produce an enzyme called beta-glucuronidase, which acts like a corrupt customs officer. It unpacks the garbage, sending estrogen back into circulation. This re-entry of estrogen creates estrogen dominance—a hormonal imbalance with symptoms such as:

- Mood swings
- Weight gain
- PMS

A fiber-rich diet acts like a traffic system, keeping everything moving smoothly toward the exit (your stool). Probiotics help by maintaining a balanced microbiome, reducing beta-glucuronidase activity. Calcium D-glucarate (CDG) can also help shuttle the estrogen metabolites out of the gut.

Calcium D-glucarate is a natural compound that supports estrogen detoxification, making it particularly beneficial for women in perimenopause who often experience estrogen dominance. CDG enhances the liver's detox pathways by promoting glucuronidation—a process where estrogen is "tagged" with glucuronic acid, preparing it for elimination through bile or urine.

Think of glucuronidation as a luggage-tagging system at an airport: CDG ensures every piece of "estrogen luggage" is tagged for disposal. CDG prevents reabsorption of estrogen in the gut by inhibiting beta-glucuronidase, an enzyme that can "rip off the tags," sending waste estrogen back into circulation. CDG acts like a vigilant recycling supervisor, ensuring estrogen waste leaves the body and doesn't clutter the system.

Why Proper Detox Pathways Matter

1. Balance Hormones: Proper detox prevents estrogen dominance, keeping hormones like progesterone, testosterone, and cortisol in check.
2. Reduce Cancer Risk: Poor detox leads to harmful estrogen metabolites (like 4-OH) accumulating, increasing DNA damage and cancer risk.
3. Promote Overall Health: Efficient detoxification supports a healthy gut, reduces inflammation, and boosts energy.

Key Support Strategies

1. Phase 1 Support:
   - Eat cruciferous vegetables (broccoli, cauliflower) for indole-3-carbinol, which favors the protective 2-OH pathway.

- Consume antioxidants like green tea, berries, and vitamin C, and consider supplements like I3C/DIM and liver support botanicals.
2. Phase 2 Support:
   - Ensure adequate intake of B vitamins, magnesium, and sulfur-rich foods (like garlic and onions).
   - Use supplements like N-acetylcysteine (NAC) or glutathione if needed.
3. Gut Support:
   - Maintain a fiber-rich diet with low-glycemic fruits, and vegetables.
   - Use probiotics to balance your gut microbiome and Calcium D-glucarate if needed.
   - Incorporate prebiotic foods and supplements such as artichokes, beets, chicory root, pomegranate, and acacia fiber.
   - Avoid processed foods and excess alcohol, which can disrupt gut health.

RECAP

1. Phase 1 (Sorting Center): Estrogen is tagged for processing, creating intermediate forms (safe, risky, or bulky).
2. Phase 2 (Packaging Plant): Tagged estrogen is wrapped up securely for disposal using enzymes powered by nutrients.
3. Gut (Shipping Depot): The packaged estrogen is sent out of the body via the stool, with the gut microbiome acting as quality control.

Why Alcohol Is Bad for the Liver and Hormones

Think of your liver as a busy office responsible for sorting out all the paperwork (metabolic tasks) that keeps your body running smoothly. Each day, it handles tasks like processing nutrients, detoxifying harmful substances, and balancing hormones like estrogen. But then, alcohol walks into the office like an urgent project with a flashing red "PRIORITY" stamp. Everything else—including managing hormones—gets shoved to the back burner while the liver scrambles to deal with this new, pressing task.

The Liver and Alcohol: A Metabolism Distraction

1. Alcohol Takes Priority:
    - Alcohol is treated like a toxic emergency by the liver. When you drink, your liver prioritizes metabolizing alcohol (turning it into less harmful substances like acetate) to prevent alcohol from poisoning the body.
    - Imagine the office manager drops all ongoing work (like hormone regulation and detoxification) to focus on a sudden, urgent task. The rest of the office's work piles up.
2. Hormones Get Neglected:
    - While the liver is metabolizing alcohol, it can't efficiently break down excess estrogen. This means estrogen levels can rise in the body, potentially disrupting hormonal balance.
    - Estrogen is like an important letter waiting to be filed. But the office is too busy with the "alcohol emergency," so the letter just sits on the desk, creating clutter and throwing off the office's efficiency.

Liver Health Supplements for Estrogen Detox

Supporting the liver is crucial for detoxifying estrogen and reducing estrogen dominance. Key supplements include:

Milk Thistle (Silymarin):
- Milk thistle supports phase I and II liver detox pathways, promoting the breakdown and elimination of hormones like estrogen.

- Acts as an antioxidant to protect liver cells from damage.
- Think of milk thistle as the city's waste processing plant, making sure estrogen is efficiently broken down.

N-Acetylcysteine (NAC):
- Increases glutathione, the liver's master antioxidant, enhancing detoxification.
- Reduces oxidative stress and supports the liver's ability to process excess hormones.

Sulforaphane (from Broccoli Sprouts):
- Activates liver enzymes that metabolize estrogen into safer, less active forms.
- Promotes healthy estrogen metabolism via the 2-hydroxyestrone pathway, reducing estrogen dominance risks.

I3C/DIM (Indole-3-Carbinol & Diindolylmethane):
- Supports healthy estrogen metabolism by promoting the conversion of estrogen into its protective 2-hydroxyestrone form, reducing estrogen dominance risks.
- Aids liver detoxification by enhancing the breakdown and elimination of excess estrogen and toxins.

Dandelion Root
- Dandelion root supports bile production and flow. Bile is essential for digesting fats and removing toxins, including excess hormones like estrogen from the body.
- Dandelion root is like a plumber who unclogs the pipes (bile ducts), ensuring that waste flows out smoothly and the house (your body) stays clean.

Turmeric (Curcumin)
- Turmeric, rich in curcumin, is a potent anti-inflammatory and antioxidant that protects liver cells from damage.

- It enhances liver detox pathways, particularly Phase 2 detoxification, which is crucial for metabolizing estrogen and other hormones.
- Turmeric is like a fire extinguisher for the liver, quelling inflammation and allowing the detoxification machinery to work safely and efficiently.

Artichoke Leaf
- Artichoke leaf is a powerhouse for stimulating bile production and protecting liver cells.
- It contains cynarin, which supports both fat digestion and toxin elimination.
- By improving bile flow, artichoke leaf helps remove excess estrogen, reducing risks of hormonal imbalances that can lead to PMS, fibroids, or estrogen-driven cancers.

Oral Contraceptive Pills and Hormones

But what if I am on birth control pills? Unfortunately, if you have been given birth control, you probably weren't given full informed consent. So many times, my female patients are on birth control because their doctor told them it would fix symptoms like heavy bleeding, migraines, or irregular periods. That is not the best approach to take. Symptoms are a gift from God to let us know something needs to be addressed!

Studies have shown that hormonal contraceptives, including oral birth control, are associated with various health risks. They can increase the risk of certain cancers, such as breast and cervical cancer. Long-term use of oral contraceptives has been linked to decreased fertility risks, with some studies suggesting a potential delay in conception after discontinuation.

> Additionally, hormonal contraceptives can impact gut health, potentially leading to an imbalance in the vaginal microbiome and increasing the risk of infections like Candida. Oral birth control also depletes the body of crucial B6, B12, folic acid, and minerals like magnesium and zinc.
>
> I was prescribed birth control in high school to "regulate" my period. Looking back, I realize I wasn't given full, informed consent or a clear explanation of the potential risks. While that experience was frustrating, it became a blessing—because now I'm able to offer my patients the informed, thoughtful guidance they deserve.

OTHER WAYS TO LOVE YOUR LIVER

1. Dry Brushing
   - How It Works: Stimulates the lymphatic system by promoting movement of lymph fluid and exfoliating the skin.
   - Benefits: Clears toxins through the lymphatic system, supports circulation, and improves skin health.
   - How to Do It: Use a natural-bristle brush to gently brush your skin in long, upward strokes toward the heart before showering.

2. Jumping on a Trampoline (Rebounding)
   - How It Works: Rebounding exercises stimulate lymphatic circulation through rhythmic movement, encouraging lymph flow and detoxification.
   - Benefits: Boosts lymphatic drainage, improves circulation, and supports cardiovascular health.
   - How to Do It: Bounce on a mini trampoline for 10–15 minutes daily.

3. Castor Oil Packs
   - How It Works: Castor oil penetrates the skin, increasing circulation and promoting lymphatic flow while supporting liver detox.
   - Benefits: Reduces inflammation, enhances lymphatic drainage, and stimulates liver detoxification.
   - How to Use It: Soak a cloth in castor oil, place it over the liver area, cover with plastic wrap, and apply heat with a hot water bottle for 20–60 minutes, or use with a castor oil pack and leave on overnight.

4. Epsom Salt Bath
   - How It Works: Epsom salts are rich in magnesium, which supports relaxation, detoxification, and healthy liver function.
   - Benefits: Can help relax muscles, draw out toxins through the skin, and reduce inflammation.
   - How to Use It: Dissolve one to two cups of Epsom salt in a warm bath and soak for 20 minutes.

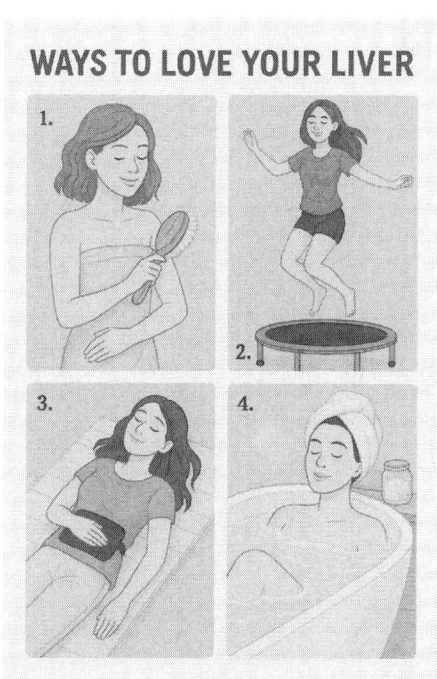

Cleansing through diet, liver health, and gentle detox practices is not about achieving perfection or following the latest trend—it's about faithfully stewarding the body God has entrusted to you, especially during the unique challenges of perimenopause. Removing processed foods, reducing toxin exposure, and embracing a gluten-free diet when needed are practical ways to support your liver so it can do the work it was designed to do. These choices help lay a foundation for clearer thinking, steadier energy, and balanced hormones at a time in life when your body is already going through profound change.

Remember Julie, who had shortened cycles? When she cut out gluten 100% and added some liver-loving herbs and botanicals to her regimen, her cycle lengthened to 26 days just by making those changes. It was difficult at first for her to go gluten free, but once she got used to it, she found it was easy. She really enjoyed taking Epsom salt baths in the evenings and using her castor oil pack at night. Rebounding is now part of her morning routine with taking supplements. Her constipation went away completely, and so did the belly bloat!

Chapter Key Takeaways:

- Look out for credible labels on food packaging such as USDA Organic, Non-GMO Project Verified, or Fair Trade.
- Gut and hormone health are impacted by the glyphosate herbicide found in our food and environment (organic and gluten-free foods are best).
- For happy hormones, focus on liver health, detoxification, and supportive supplements.

CHAPTER 5

Connect to Your Endocrine Signals

> So we fasted and petitioned our God about this,
> and he answered our prayer.
>
> —Ezra 8:21 (NIV)

My patient Mary was having a difficult time losing weight. Twenty pounds had crept on during perimenopause, and she was frustrated! She decided to go with the new diet she heard about on social media: intermittent fasting, or IF. She was shocked when she gained ten pounds as a result. I told her not to get frustrated, because we would figure it out. First, we started talking about gut health and how to cleanse her environment, and then I had her wear a continuous glucose monitor (CGM). She was spiking her blood sugar in the morning when she wasn't eating. For her, she couldn't intermittent fast daily, especially not during her luteal phase. Changing her diet to starting the day with healthy fats and protein got her back on track. She lost 12 pounds in the first two months.

Connect to Fasting for Your Health

Yes, it might seem uncomfortable to think of fasting. It's like a muscle: you have to flex the fasting muscle to get better at it. You are not going to just jump into a 48-hour fast. You will start by setting the clock back on your eating window slowly. But ladies, we need to do things a little differently during perimenopause to support our hormones.

Let's explain insulin resistance first. Think of insulin as a popular song that plays to get your cells' attention. Its job is to let your cells know that glucose (sugar) is in the bloodstream and needs to be taken up for energy. Normally, your cells "listen" to the song and respond by opening their doors to let glucose in.

Imagine the first time you hear this song. It's catchy, and every time it plays, you notice it immediately. Your cells are like enthusiastic listeners who respond by dancing (absorbing glucose) and using it for energy. This is how a healthy body processes insulin signals efficiently.

But then, you start hearing this song everywhere. It's on the radio at home, playing in the car, and blasting at the gym. Every meal, every snack, every sugary drink triggers the release of insulin—playing that same song over and over again. Over time, it becomes so familiar that you barely notice it anymore.

Now you're in the grocery store, and the song comes on in the background. Do you pay attention to it? Probably not. It's faded into the noise. Similarly, your cells stop responding to insulin as they once did because they've been overexposed to it. They don't "open their doors" as effectively to glucose anymore.

What Happens Next?

- Since your cells aren't responding, glucose stays in the bloodstream longer, causing high blood sugar levels.

- The pancreas, like a desperate DJ, turns up the volume, pumping out even more insulin to try to get the cells' attention.
- Over time, this overproduction of insulin exhausts the pancreas and can lead to type 2 diabetes.
- Chronic high blood sugar creates inflammation throughout the body, damaging blood vessels, nerve endings, and organs. This systemic inflammation contributes to fatigue, hormonal imbalance, brain fog, and increased risk of heart disease and autoimmune flares.

Just like you become numb to a song you've heard too many times, your cells become numb to insulin when it's constantly present. This is insulin resistance—a condition where the signals are there, but your body stops paying attention. Breaking this cycle involves "changing the station" by adopting healthier habits such as balancing your meals, exercising, and managing stress, helping your cells tune back into the message.

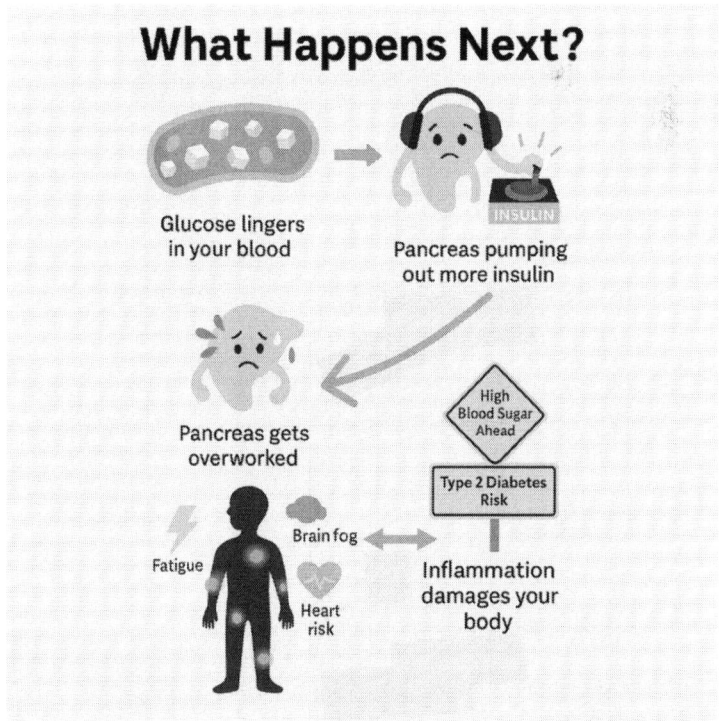

Fasting Options

12-Hour Fast
- Glycogen Depletion: Liver glycogen stores (your stored form of sugar) begin to deplete, prompting a mild metabolic shift.
- Blood Sugar Regulation: Early improvements in insulin sensitivity (your body starts responding better to insulin).
- Cellular Repair: The initiation of autophagy (cell cleanup and recycling of old parts) starts in some cells.

16-Hour Fast (Intermittent Fasting)
- Enhanced Fat Burning: Lipolysis increases (your body starts breaking down fat for energy).
- Improved Mental Clarity: Ketone production begins, which fuels the brain.
- Hormonal Balance: Growth hormone secretion increases, aiding muscle repair and fat metabolism.

24-Hour Fast
- Deepened Autophagy: More cellular repair and waste removal.
- Reduction in Inflammation: Pro-inflammatory cytokines like IL-6 may decrease.
- Metabolic Reset: Notable improvements in insulin sensitivity and glucose regulation.

36-48 Hour Fast
- Ketosis: Deeper reliance on fat and ketones (fat-derived fuel) as primary energy sources.
- Immune System Reset: Damaged immune cells begin to be cleared through autophagy.

- Gut Healing: Mucosal lining repair and reduced gut inflammation; digestion gets a rest.

72-Hour Fast
- Cellular Rejuvenation: Enhanced autophagy, particularly in immune cells and mitochondria (energy factories in cells).
- Immune System Regeneration and Anti-Aging Benefits: Stem cells begin repopulating the immune system (as shown in animal and some human data).

5+ Days (Prolonged Fast)
- Maximum Autophagy: Significant cellular repair and renewal.
- Stem Cell Activation: High levels of stem cell production for tissue repair.
- Chronic Disease Mitigation: Positive impact on insulin resistance, blood pressure, and inflammation (under medical supervision).

Key Considerations
- Always prioritize water, electrolytes, and proper mineral balance. Check out my favorite electrolytes in the resources.
- Prolonged fasting beyond 48 hours should be supervised, especially for those with medical conditions.
- Break the fast with nutrient-dense foods, prioritizing healthy fats, proteins, and complex carbs. Avoid refined sugars and processed foods, which can spike insulin and inflammatory markers.

Fasting has been shown to positively influence various hormonal pathways, leading to improved metabolic health. Intermittent fasting (IF) enhances insulin sensitivity, allowing cells to utilize glucose more effectively, thereby reducing blood sugar levels and the risk of type 2 diabetes.

Weight loss achieved through fasting can lead to a reduction in adipose tissue, which is a significant site for estrogen production. This decrease in fat mass can help lower circulating estrogen levels, potentially reducing the risk of estrogen-dependent conditions.

Fasting for women in perimenopause should be done at the right time, or you are not only setting yourself up for heartache, but you can also impact your cortisol levels. The best time is going to be that first half of your cycle, the follicular phase.

Why Fasting Is Beneficial in the Follicular Phase

The follicular phase, the first half of the menstrual cycle from the start of menstruation to ovulation, is characterized by rising estrogen levels and lower progesterone. Fasting during this phase can be more effective and better tolerated for hormonal balance due to the body's improved resilience to metabolic stress.

Insulin Sensitivity Is Higher: During the follicular phase, estrogen levels rise, enhancing insulin sensitivity. This makes fasting more effective for blood sugar regulation and fat metabolism. Women with PCOS, who often have insulin resistance, can particularly benefit from fasting during this phase to reduce insulin spikes and improve metabolic health.

Reduced Cortisol Sensitivity: The body is generally more resilient to stress in the follicular phase compared to the luteal phase, where progesterone peaks and cortisol sensitivity increases. This makes short fasting windows (12-16 hours) safer and less likely to disrupt adrenal function.

Mitigates Estrogen Dominance: Fasting can reduce inflammation and optimize liver function, aiding in the metabolism of excess estrogen. This is beneficial for conditions like estrogen dominance or PCOS.

Why Avoid Fasting in the Luteal Phase?

A common mistake I see among perimenopausal women is fasting during the luteal phase, and their progesterone is what pays the price. I often say, "Protect the progesterone!"

- Progesterone rises post-ovulation, increasing hunger and sensitivity to stress.
- The body is better suited to nutrient-rich, frequent meals during this phase.

Incorporate Hormone-Supporting Supplements:

- Magnesium: Modulates the HPA axis (hypothalamic-pituitary-adrenal, a stress response system) by dampening excitatory neurotransmission (overactive nerve signaling). This helps regulate cortisol output and reduce stress-induced hormonal dysregulation (imbalances in hormone levels caused by chronic stress).
- B Vitamins (B6, B12, Folate): Essential cofactors for steroid hormone biosynthesis (the production of hormones like estrogen and progesterone from cholesterol) and for methylation pathways that detoxify estrogen metabolites, supporting balanced estrogen-progesterone dynamics.
- Adaptogens (e.g., Ashwagandha, Rhodiola): Enhance the body's resilience to physical and psychological stress by regulating HPA axis activity and supporting adrenal homeostasis.
- Omega-3 Fatty Acids: Exert anti-inflammatory effects and maintain neuronal membrane fluidity (how flexible the outer layer of a nerve cell is), supporting both brain function and hormone receptor sensitivity.

Healthy Fasting Practices:

- Stay Hydrated: Drink water infused with electrolytes or herbal teas to maintain energy and hydration.

- Light Exercise: Pair fasting with activities like mobility training, walking, or strength training to support metabolic health without excessive stress. This means no HIIT training or sprints.

Incorporate Hormone-Supporting Supplements

- Magnesium: This is the "calm-down mineral," which regulates stress and supports the adrenal glands.
- B Vitamins (B6, B12, Folate): "Craftsmen" that build estrogen and progesterone balance.
- Adaptogens (e.g., Ashwagandha, Rhodiola): The "stress whisperers," which help manage cortisol.
- Omega-3 Fatty Acids: These are the "firefighters" that reduce inflammation and promote hormonal health.

What About Coffee on an Empty Stomach?

Consuming coffee on an empty stomach is a topic of considerable interest, particularly regarding its effects on metabolism and overall health. The impact of coffee consumption, especially caffeinated coffee, can vary depending on individual health conditions and preferences. Many people enjoy adding medium-chain triglyceride (MCT) oil and butter to their coffee (my favorite!), which can provide a source of healthy fats that may help sustain energy levels during fasting periods.

Research indicates that coffee, particularly caffeinated varieties, can have both beneficial and adverse effects on metabolic health. For instance, studies have shown that coffee consumption can lead to acute changes in glucose metabolism. A study by Yarmolinsky et al. found that both caffeinated and decaffeinated coffee can decrease levels of glucose-dependent insulinotropic peptide (GIP)—a hormone produced in the gut, which helps the body release insulin after eating, playing a crucial role in insulin secretion. This suggests that coffee may have a role in modulating insulin sensitivity, although the acute effects of caffeine can sometimes impair glucose tolerance temporarily.

When consumed on an empty stomach, caffeine can stimulate the adrenal glands, leading to increased cortisol production. This response can be likened to a "fight or flight" reaction, where the body prepares for immediate energy expenditure. While this can enhance alertness and focus, it may also lead to increased stress levels if the body is not in a balanced state. Thus, for individuals sensitive to caffeine, consuming it on an empty stomach could potentially exacerbate feelings of anxiety or stress. Adding fats like MCT oil or butter to coffee may help buffer the adrenal response by providing a more stable source of energy and reducing the cortisol spike typically triggered by caffeine alone.

MCT oil provides a quick source of energy that can help stabilize blood sugar levels, which is particularly beneficial during fasting. This combination can create a more balanced metabolic environment, allowing for sustained energy without the sharp spikes and crashes associated with high-carb breakfasts. The fats in MCT oil and butter can also promote satiety, helping to curb hunger during fasting periods.

An analogy to illustrate this concept is to think of coffee as a high-octane fuel for a race car. While it can provide a powerful boost in performance, if the engine (your body) is not adequately prepared, it may lead to overheating (stress) or even damage (adrenal fatigue). However, by adding MCT oil and butter, you are essentially adding a stabilizing agent to the fuel, allowing the engine to run smoothly and efficiently without the risk of overheating.

My take: While drinking coffee on an empty stomach can have both positive and negative effects, the addition of healthy fats can enhance its benefits and reduce potential stress on the body. If having caffeinated coffee in the morning, add butter and MCT oil.

> So we do not focus on what is seen, but on what is unseen. For what is seen is temporary, but what is unseen is eternal.
>
> —2 Corinthians 4:18 (CSB)

This chapter may feel overwhelming—I understand. But just like the verse reminds us, true transformation often happens where we can't see it. These choices may not produce instant results, but they're building something lasting beneath the surface. Trust that the inner work matters, even when it's invisible. Stay faithful to the process.

Benefits of Continuous Glucose Monitors

A continuous glucose monitor (CGM) is a wearable device that tracks glucose levels in real time throughout the day and night by measuring sugar in the fluid just beneath the skin. Wearing a CGM is going to change how you eat food.

Did you know your mood can be affected by your blood sugar? Going on a blood sugar roller coaster can really be an issue. When your blood sugar shoots up quickly from a sugary or carb-heavy meal, insulin overshoots, and your blood sugar can bottom out. Then you eat to feel better, and it goes up again.

A continuous glucose monitor provides real-time data about your blood glucose levels, enabling precise insights into how fasting, diet, exercise, and hormonal changes affect your metabolism. For women in perimenopause, a CGM is particularly beneficial due to the metabolic shifts driven by fluctuating estrogen and progesterone levels.

How a CGM Helps

- Tracks daily glucose patterns, revealing how your body handles food intake at different hormonal phases.
- Identifies times when fasting might be more effective, or when additional nutritional support is needed to stabilize blood sugar.

Think of a CGM as a compass for your metabolic journey during perimenopause. It guides you through fluctuating hormonal landscapes, helping you avoid metabolic "storms."

- Tracks daily glucose patterns, revealing how your body handles food intake at different hormonal phases.
- Identifies times when fasting might be more effective, or when additional nutritional support is needed to stabilize blood sugar.

Think of a CGM as a compass for your metabolic journey during perimenopause. It guides you through fluctuating hormonal landscapes, helping you avoid metabolic "storms."

Using CGM Insights to Fine-Tune

- Meal Timing:
  - Experiment with a longer fasting window (e.g., 16:8) if glucose is stable.
  - If glucose dips or spikes too much, shorten the fasting window.
- Macronutrient Balance:
  - Adjust protein, fat, or carb ratios based on which meals keep glucose most stable.
- Lifestyle Factors:
  - Note how stress, sleep, and hydration impact glucose trends.
  - Address these areas if patterns suggest cortisol-driven spikes or dips.

- Patterns During Exercise:
  - Strength training can cause a temporary rise in glucose due to adrenaline release—a normal, adaptive response that reflects hormesis, where short-term stress leads to long-term resilience and metabolic health gains.
  - Cardio or walking after meals should help lower post-meal spikes. This is helpful to decrease harmful glucose spikes.

STEPS TO HARMONIZING GLUCOSE LEVELS

Remember the analogy: Insulin resistance is like hearing a song so many times—at home, in the car, on the radio—that your brain starts to ignore it. Your cells, much like you in the grocery store, stop "listening" to insulin's message to absorb glucose. To fix this, we need to "change the station," introducing fresh signals and rhythms to reset your cells' attention. Here's how:

Step 1: Start with Protein and Healthy Fats (A New Playlist)

- Why It Helps: Protein and fats introduce a new "sound" to your cells. They don't cause the loud glucose and insulin spikes that overwhelm your system. Instead, they stabilize blood sugar and restore balance.
- How to Do It: Begin every meal with animal-based protein and healthy fats.
  - Example: Start your day with eggs cooked in grassfed butter and avocado on the side.
- Think of this as playing a calming, steady beat instead of the loud, repetitive chorus that glucose spikes represent.

Step 2: Incorporate Low-Oxalate Veggies (Fresh Lyrics)

- Why It Helps: Vegetables such as broccoli or cauliflower that feature minimal anti-nutrients provide fiber and nutrients without disrupting the flow of energy in your body.

- How to Do It: Pair these veggies with protein and fats to enhance absorption.
  - Example: Pair grilled chicken thighs with roasted cauliflower and olive oil.
- These veggies are like thoughtful new lyrics that complement the rhythm of your meal.

Step 3: Apple Cider Vinegar Before Meals (Tuning the Station)

- Why It Helps: Apple cider vinegar lowers the "volume" of glucose spikes after meals by improving insulin sensitivity.
- How to Do It: Mix 1–2 tablespoons in water and drink before eating.
- ACV is like adjusting the bass and treble on your radio—softening the harsh spikes and enhancing the overall harmony.

Step 4: Berberine as a Glucose Coach

- Why It Helps: Berberine amplifies your cells' ability to listen to insulin, effectively making them "re-tune" to its message.
- How to Do It: Take 500 mg of berberine with meals, especially when consuming carbs.
- Berberine is like a DJ, ensuring the music (insulin signaling) plays at the perfect level for your cells to respond.

Step 5: Weightlifting and Building Muscle (Adding New Instruments)

- Why It Helps: Building muscle increases glucose storage capacity, making your body more responsive to insulin.
- How to Do It: Lift weights two to four times per week, focusing on compound movements like squats and deadlifts. Lift heavy, ladies!
- Muscle is like adding new instruments to your metabolic "band"—each one helps handle glucose, creating a fuller, more balanced sound.

Step 6: Walk After Meals (Dynamic Transitions in the Song)

- Why It Helps: Walking after eating lowers glucose spikes by using muscles to absorb sugar directly.
- How to Do It: Take a 10–15-minute walk within 30 minutes of eating.
- Walking is like adding a smooth transition between verses in a song, keeping the energy steady and preventing abrupt spikes or crashes.

Step 7: Save Dessert or Carbs for Last (The Encore)

- Why It Helps: Eating carbs after protein, fats, and fiber slows their absorption, reducing the insulin surge.
- How to Do It: Finish meals with a small portion of carbs or dessert rather than eating them alone.
  - Example: Start with steak and veggies, then enjoy a square of dark chocolate.
- Carbs at the end are like a crowd-pleasing encore that doesn't disrupt the concert flow but leaves you satisfied.

Step 8: Spacing Meals (Adjusting the Playlist Order)

- Why It Helps: Longer breaks between meals give your body time to process glucose and lower insulin levels, while also activating the migrating motor complex—a digestive "cleansing wave" that helps clear out bacteria and food debris, supporting gut health and reducing bloating.
- How to Do It: Space meals four to six hours apart and consider a time-restricted eating window (e.g., eight hours).
- Meal spacing is like curating the perfect playlist—you don't want the same song on repeat; you need breaks to appreciate the music.

Step 9: Hydration and Sleep (Silent Interludes)

- Hydration: Drinking water keeps your metabolism running smoothly, like keeping the radio free of static.
    - Add a pinch of sea salt for electrolytes if fasting or sweating heavily. Test your electrolyte drinks with your CGM if you are using them with fasting. Make sure they are not causing a spike in your glucose!
- Sleep: Poor sleep disrupts insulin sensitivity, so aim for seven to nine hours nightly.
    - Create a calming bedtime routine to tune out the day's noise.
- Hydration and sleep are like silent interludes in your playlist—they allow for recovery and reset before the next track.

Step 10: Manage Stress (Avoid Commercial Breaks)

- Why It Helps: Chronic stress is like a loud, jarring commercial interrupting your playlist—it raises cortisol and glucose.
- How to Do It: Practice prayerful meditation and deep breathing exercises to keep stress in check. Adaptogens can also help.
- Managing stress ensures your playlist flows seamlessly without annoying interruptions.

Step 11: Use a CGM to Fine-Tune

- Why It Helps: A continuous glucose monitor lets you see how your blood sugar responds to meals, exercise, and lifestyle changes in real-time.
- How to Do It: Track your patterns and adjust based on the data.
    - Example: If you notice glucose spikes after certain meals, tweak ingredients or portion sizes. A peak can also mean a food sensitivity or intolerance.
- A CGM is like having a sound engineer fine-tuning the balance of your metabolic "mix."

Changing the Station Recap

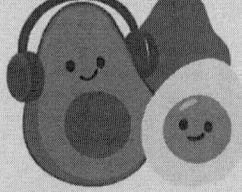

Protein and Fat
The steady rhythm of your metabolic playlist.

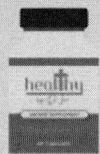 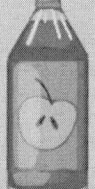

ACV and Berberine
Fine-tune insulin signaling.

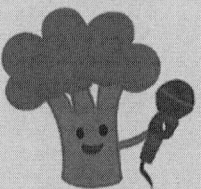

Low-Oxalate Veggies
Fresh, complementary lyrics

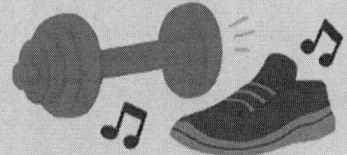

Weightlifting and Walking
Add new instruments and smooth transitions

Dessert Last

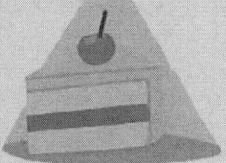

Save the encore
for a balanced finale

Meal Spacing, Hydration, and Sleep
Provide interludes for recovery

Stress Management
Avoid jarring interruptions in your metabolic flow

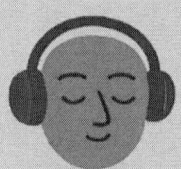 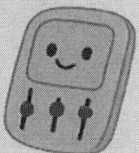

CGM Tracking
The engineer ensuring that your station plays at its best.

CHANGING THE STATION RECAP

- Protein and Fat: The steady rhythm of your metabolic playlist.
- Low-Oxalate Veggies: Fresh, complementary lyrics.
- ACV and Berberine: Fine-tune the volume and clarity of insulin signaling.
- Weightlifting and Walking: Add new instruments and smooth transitions.
- Dessert Last: Save the encore for a balanced finale.
- Meal Spacing, Hydration, and Sleep: Provide interludes for recovery.
- Stress Management: Avoid jarring interruptions in your metabolic flow.
- CGM Tracking: The engineer ensuring that your station plays at its best.

By implementing these strategies, you're essentially "changing the station" on your body's metabolic habits. Instead of constant noise and overexposure to insulin, you're creating a balanced, harmonious playlist that your cells can hear, respond to, and thrive on.

WHY DOES THIS MATTER?

Because trying to lose weight while in a state of insulin resistance is like turning up the volume on a broken speaker. No matter how "loud" your efforts—cutting calories, exercising more—your cells can't hear the signal. The body remains locked in fat-storage mode, prioritizing blood sugar regulation over fat burning. This can be so frustrating. I hear it from my perimenopause patients all the time: "I have tried everything and can't lose weight!"

Studies confirm this metabolic blockade. In a pivotal review published in *The Lancet* (2022), researchers concluded that insulin resistance impairs the ability of fat cells to release energy, making weight loss significantly harder—even with diet and exercise. Another study from *Cell Metabolism* showed that chronically elevated insulin levels blunt lipolysis, the process of breaking down stored fat.

Until insulin sensitivity is restored—through strategies like balancing meals, strength training, fasting appropriately, and managing stress—the body resists weight loss, even when the math "should" work.

Weighted Vests: A Tool for Perimenopause

Walking with a weighted vest offers multiple health benefits, including increased calorie burn, enhanced cardiovascular fitness, improved bone density, and muscle strengthening. Adding extra weight during walking requires more energy expenditure, leading to higher caloric burn compared to regular walking.

Studies show that this additional resistance challenges the cardiovascular system, potentially improving heart and lung capacity over time. One of the most significant benefits is its effect on bone health, as the increased mechanical loading on bones can help stimulate bone formation and reduce the risk of osteoporosis.

Additionally, walking with added weight engages lower body and core muscles, leading to increased muscle strength, endurance, and better balance, which may lower the risk of falls.

Despite its benefits, using a weighted vest improperly can lead to joint stress, postural issues, or injury if the weight is too heavy or distributed unevenly. Extra weight can place additional strain on the knees, hips, and lower back, particularly for individuals with preexisting conditions such as arthritis or back pain.

Choosing the appropriate vest weight is crucial for safety and effectiveness. Experts recommend starting with a vest that is 5–10% of your body weight and gradually increasing as your strength and endurance improve. For example, a person weighing 150 pounds should start with a 7.5 to 15-pound vest.

Listening to your body is key—if discomfort or pain arises, it's best to reduce the weight or adjust usage. The vest should fit snugly and distribute weight evenly to prevent shifting, which could lead to imbalance or muscle strain.

Peptides for Perimenopause: What About GLP-1s?

GLP-1s (Glucagon-like Peptide-1 receptor agonists) are medications that mimic a naturally occurring hormone involved in blood sugar regulation and appetite control. These drugs are primarily used to treat type 2 diabetes but are increasingly being studied for weight loss and metabolic health, making them a potential tool for managing blood sugar during perimenopause.

How GLP-1s Work

GLP-1 is a hormone released in response to food intake that plays several roles:

1. Enhances Insulin Secretion: GLP-1 stimulates the pancreas to release insulin in response to elevated blood glucose.
2. Suppresses Glucagon: It reduces glucagon (a hormone that raises blood sugar) production, helping keep glucose levels stable.
3. Slows Gastric Emptying: It delays the stomach's emptying of food into the small intestine, leading to a slower rise in blood sugar.
4. Reduces Appetite: GLP-1 acts on the brain to promote feelings of fullness, reducing calorie intake.
5. Reduces Inflammation: GLP-1s modulate inflammatory signaling pathways (like NF-κB) and lower levels of pro-inflammatory cytokines like IL-6 and TNF-alpha, which are chemicals that drive inflammation in the body.
6. Supports Brain Health: GLP-1 receptors are present in the brain and are associated with neuroprotection, enhanced cognitive function, and reduced risk of neurodegenerative processes.

Think of GLP-1 as the conductor of an orchestra—it ensures that insulin, glucagon, and appetite signals work in harmony to maintain metabolic balance.

Benefits of GLP-1s for Perimenopause

1. Improved Insulin Sensitivity
   Hormonal fluctuations—particularly estrogen decline—can impair glucose regulation. GLP-1s enhance the insulin response and reduce insulin resistance, helping rebalance metabolism.
2. Weight Management
   Perimenopausal weight gain, especially abdominal fat, is driven by shifts in hormones and stress. GLP-1s reduce hunger and food intake, supporting gradual and sustainable fat loss.
3. Blood Sugar Stability
   By smoothing out glucose spikes and troughs, GLP-1s help prevent energy crashes, cravings, and mood swings often linked to blood sugar fluctuations.
4. Cardiovascular Benefits
   Perimenopause increases the risk of cardiovascular disease. GLP-1s have been shown to lower cholesterol and reduce inflammation, benefiting heart health.
5. Reduced Inflammation
   Chronic low-grade inflammation often increases in perimenopause. GLP-1s help calm inflammatory pathways that contribute to metabolic dysfunction and mood disturbances.
6. Cognitive and Mood Support
   With GLP-1 receptor activity in the brain, these medications show promise for supporting memory, improving mood, and potentially protecting against neurodegenerative changes often accelerated by hormonal shifts.

How GLP-1s Align with Your Blood Sugar Strategy

If you're already focused on:

- Protein and Healthy Fats: GLP-1s complement this by optimizing how your body processes the food you eat.

- Low-Oxalate Veggies and Fiber: GLP-1s amplify the glucose-stabilizing effects of fiber-rich meals.
- Apple Cider Vinegar and Berberine: These hacks work synergistically with GLP-1s to improve insulin sensitivity.
- Weightlifting and Walking: Exercise helps increase your muscle's ability to use glucose, while GLP-1s improve the hormonal regulation of blood sugar.

Analogy: GLP-1s are like adding a high-tech autopilot to your metabolic "station reset." They enhance and automate many of the manual strategies you're already using. I use this strategy with select patients and use microdosing often to help with inflammatory processes. GLP-1s do have side effects and risks. Consult your integrative physician to learn more and ask about whether GLP-1s are right for you.

Examples of GLP-1 Medications:

Semaglutide (Ozempic, Wegovy): GLP-1 agonist
Tirzepatide (Mounjaro): Dual GLP-1 and GIP agonist
Retatrutide: Triple-hormone receptor agonist

As you consider tools like continuous glucose monitoring, GLP-1 medications, and fasting, remember that these are not just health strategies—they are opportunities to steward your body with wisdom and intention. By aligning your habits with God's design for nourishment, rest, and balance, you create space for healing and resilience, even in the hormonal shifts of perimenopause. With His guidance, you can build practices that support steady energy, clear thinking, and vibrant health to better serve the purpose He has for your life.

Remember Mary—the patient who was intermittent fasting every day before she came to see me—who was gaining weight? She was getting so frustrated since she was doing all the things. We decided at the first appointment to put on a CGM and see what was going on. It turned out that she was spiking in the morning. It was a stress response to chronic prolonged intermittent fasting! We adjusted her to a 12-hour overnight fast with a protein-packed breakfast. Adding in weightlifting made her metabolic flexible, and she lost the weight, had more energy, and felt like herself again!

Chapter Key Takeaways:

- Fasting during the follicular phase is ideal and most effective for hormonal balance
- Commit to strategies, such as wearing a CGM, for enhancing your body's metabolic habits
- GLP-1s are a tool that have benefits (e.g., weight loss, blood sugar balance, heart health) for perimenopause

CHAPTER 6

Cultivate Strength

> Don't be wise in your own eyes; fear the Lord
> and turn away from evil. This will be healing for
> your body and strengthening to your bones.
>
> —Proverbs 3: 7–8 (CSB)

When we walk in humility and follow God's word, it brings true healing. Cultivate healthy practices to build strength, nourish yourself deeply, and reconnect with your health—as an act of obedience and care for the life and temple God has entrusted to you.

My patient Ada decided at age 39 to run a full marathon. Pretty awesome, right? What a goal! Unfortunately, she came to me after she completed the marathon and had gained 20 pounds. She gained weight during her training for a marathon while running 26 miles. How awful, right? She not only burnt herself out, but she also damaged her adrenals and her hormones.

It was time to take back her health. Ada didn't have regrets, but, looking back, she realized she had put a lot of strain on her body. Not only was she training for the marathon, but she was also working part time, home schooling her kids, and of course being a wife. Phew!

The only thing I probably wouldn't recommend to a perimenopausal women is training for a marathon. It may be possible to train for a half marathon, if you time it correctly with your cycle and lift weights while doing it.

The good news is that, with focus on syncing her cycle (more on this in the 28-day plan) and supporting adrenal health, Ada was able to get back on track, lose weight, and get her hormones under control again. Keep in mind that it can take up to a year to recover extremely fatigued adrenals.

We lose muscle as we age, but did you know that in perimenopause we can take action to slow down this process?

Hormonal Shifts: A Factory for Muscle Health

Estrogen and testosterone are like the managers of a muscle factory, keeping operations efficient and productive. Estrogen supports muscle repair, recovery, and inflammation control, while testosterone promotes protein synthesis and strength. When both decline during perimenopause, the factory loses its leadership—slowing muscle maintenance, reducing strength, and increasing the risk of muscle loss.

DHEA, made mostly in your adrenal glands, is a building block hormone that your body can turn into other hormones—like testosterone or estrogen—by moving it down the hormone pathway, depending on what your body needs. It boosts energy production in the factory by supporting mitochondrial function and reducing inflammation, making the environment more conducive to muscle repair.

Levels of DHEA drop with age, starting in your 30s and accelerating during perimenopause. With less DHEA available, the factory loses flexibility and adaptability in hormone production, leading to inefficiencies in muscle repair and growth.

Pregnenolone is like the resource coordinator in the factory, responsible for distributing raw materials to different departments. It's the "mother hormone" used to produce other key hormones like progesterone, cortisol, DHEA, estrogen, and testosterone.

Aging reduces pregnenolone production, which creates a resource bottleneck in the factory. With fewer resources to go around, the production of critical hormones (like estrogen and testosterone) slows.

Progesterone's role in the factory is like the stress management supervisor, ensuring workers stay calm and productive under pressure. Progesterone balances the effects of cortisol, which can break down muscle tissue when levels are too high. It helps promote restful sleep, which is crucial for muscle recovery and repair. Have you noticed in perimenopause that your sleep isn't as good?

Progesterone is one of the first hormones to drop during perimenopause, leading to poor stress regulation and increased cortisol levels. Higher cortisol from reduced progesterone disrupts protein synthesis and accelerates muscle breakdown, like stressed-out workers making mistakes or quitting their jobs.

Hormonal Shifts: Disruption in the Factory

- The decline in estrogen, testosterone, DHEA, pregnenolone, and progesterone creates a cascading leadership crisis in the factory.
- Muscle repair slows down due to less oversight and fewer resources.

Stress (cortisol) becomes harder to manage, creating a chaotic work environment.

Protein Turnover Becomes Less Efficient: Supply Chain Strain

- Pregnenolone and DHEA shortages reduce the supply of resources for protein synthesis. The factory can't replenish lost materials quickly, leading to a steady decline in muscle mass.

Decreased Physical Activity: Worker Burnout

- Reduced DHEA and progesterone levels cause fatigue and make stress harder to manage, reducing motivation for physical activity.
- Inactivity leads to weaker muscles and fewer signals to preserve mass.

Increased Fat Mass: Storage Overflow

- With less progesterone and DHEA to balance cortisol, fat accumulates, cluttering the factory.
- Chronic inflammation from fat mass further disrupts operations.

Changes in Mitochondria: Energy Blackouts

- Lower DHEA and pregnenolone contribute to mitochondrial dysfunction, reducing energy production.
- Energy shortages slow muscle repair and growth processes.

Loss of Neuromuscular Connections: Broken Communication Lines

- Progesterone declines weaken the connections between nerves and muscles, causing miscommunication.
- Muscles shrink from lack of stimulation, like workers who stop showing up because they're not receiving orders.

Cultivate a Balance of Hormones

Low estrogen levels during perimenopause occur due to natural changes in the body as a woman transitions to menopause. Perimenopause is characterized by fluctuations in hormone production, particularly of estrogens and progesterone, as ovarian function begins to decline. The absence of ovulation (anovulatory cycles) also disrupts the balance between estrogen and progesterone, which can lead to periods of both low and high estrogen. The key during this transition is to support progesterone, which plays a vital role in counterbalancing estrogen, calming the nervous system, stabilizing mood, and supporting sleep. Without sufficient progesterone, even normal estrogen levels can feel overwhelming, and the overall hormonal rhythm becomes more chaotic.

Chronic stress can lead to an increase in cortisol, the body's stress hormone. Elevated cortisol levels can disrupt the hypothalamic-pituitary-ovarian (HPO) axis, which regulates reproductive hormones, reducing estrogen production. Think of the HPO axis as a computer system that synchronizes a chain reaction between the brain (signals hormone production) and ovaries—helping to control the menstrual cycle and fertility. Contributing factors:

- Poor sleep (e.g., due to hot flashes or night sweats)
- Poor nutrition or calorie restriction
- Blood sugar dysregulation
- Excessive exercise
- Adipose tissue converts androgens (produced by the adrenal glands) into estrone, a weaker form of estrogen

Progesterone and estrogen work like a seesaw. When one side starts dipping too much, the balance is thrown off, leading to periods of low estrogen. When progesterone levels drop, estrogen's effects can become more pronounced, leading to symptoms associated with estrogen dominance.

Progesterone's influence on estrogen receptors and its modulation of estrogen activity can also affect how much functional estrogen is available. Progesterone can regulate the expression of estrogen receptors on target tissues, influencing how sensitive those tissues are to estrogen. This modulation impacts the availability of functional estrogen, even if serum estrogen levels appear normal.

Estrogen and Progesterone: The Seesaw of Balance

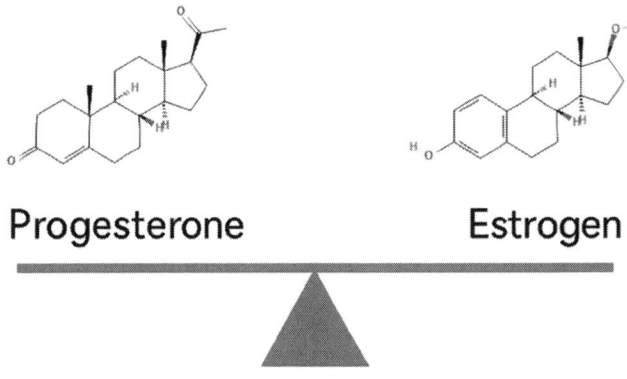

Low progesterone:

- Estrogen becomes dominant
- More estrogen receptors active

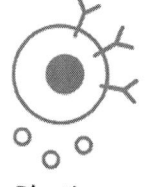

Bloating

Symptoms worsen

Mood swings

Breast tenderness

Even normal estrogen levels can feel too high when progesterone drops.

UNDERSTANDING ESTROGEN DOMINANCE: RECAP

Estrogen dominance occurs when estrogen levels are too high relative to progesterone. This imbalance can happen even if estrogen levels are normal, but progesterone levels are low, which is common during perimenopause.

- Why It Happens in Perimenopause:
  - Progesterone production drops as ovulation becomes irregular, while estrogen may still fluctuate wildly
  - Environmental xenoestrogens (found in plastics, pesticides, and personal care products) can amplify estrogenic effects
  - Poor liver detoxification or gut health may prevent estrogen from being properly broken down and eliminated
- Symptoms of Estrogen Dominance:
  - Heavy or irregular periods
  - Breast tenderness
  - Bloating and weight gain, especially around the abdomen
  - Mood swings, irritability, or anxiety

What about Medical or Surgical Factors?

- Conditions and interventions:
  - Hysterectomy with oophorectomy: Removal of the ovaries leads to an immediate and significant drop in estrogen production.
  - Certain medications: Treatments like aromatase inhibitors (used in breast cancer) block estrogen production.
  - Autoimmune disorders: Conditions like autoimmune thyroid disease or premature ovarian insufficiency (POI means that ovaries stop working normally) can impair ovarian function.
  - If the ovaries are surgically removed, it's like shutting down the hormone factory altogether, leading to low to no production of estrogen and progesterone.

Optimize Hormonal Balance

Certain herbs can help, but sometimes bioidentical hormones are needed.

- DHEA Supplements: May help restore levels and improve energy, muscle repair, and hormonal flexibility.
- Pregnenolone Supplements: Can boost the availability of precursor hormones and reduce stress-related cortisol imbalances.
- Progesterone Therapy: Supports sleep, helps downregulate cortisol output, and helps regulate inflammation.

Test, don't guess. Always check with a healthcare provider to evaluate your hormone levels and determine the right supplementation or therapy.

How to Test Hormones!

Serum vs. Blood Spot:
While testing endogenous (naturally produced in your body) hormones in serum or blood spot reveals the same levels, assessing topical hormone supplementation with serum testing grossly underestimates the amount of hormone being delivered to tissues. Blood spot tests blood in the capillary beds (arterial/venous/lymphatic) from the finger, and thus better reflects tissue hormone levels.

Serum vs. Saliva:
With saliva measuring the bioavailable (non-protein-bound) fraction of circulating hormones that can freely diffuse into tissues, it provides a more accurate assessment of topical hormone supplementation than serum. Serum levels do not rise significantly after topical dosing. By contrast, saliva levels do—reflecting tissue delivery of the topically delivered hormone.

Blood Spot/Saliva vs. Urine:
Urine testing cannot accurately assess topical or oral medications as it is not reflective of tissue uptake, and it may show no uptake with topical or extremely high levels with oral medications. Urine testing is not recommended for assessing vaginal hormone delivery as there is a high risk of contamination of the urine sample leading to false-high results. Understanding your urine metabolites is a great way to access how your body is breaking down estrogens.

Saliva testing is my favorite to provide the best assessment of oral, topical, and vaginal hormone supplementation.

Building Muscle During Perimenopause

Building muscle in this phase of life requires a strategic combination of nutrition, supplementation, and exercise tailored to counteract hormonal changes.

LIFTING WEIGHTS

How should we be moving our bodies during perimenopause? How should we link it to our cycle?

What we should avoid during a health crisis is pushing our bodies with high-intensity interval training (HIIT) or long-distance endurance workouts.

By "health crisis," I mean when you're experiencing persistent symptoms or have a diagnosed condition like autoimmune diseases (e.g., Graves' or Hashimoto's), irregular menstrual cycles, chronic headaches, bloating, or digestive issues.

These symptoms aren't just annoyances—they're God-given signals that something in your body needs attention. Pushing harder in this state can worsen the imbalance rather than support healing.

Regarding perimenopause and cardio: I am not a fan of splat points; this is where at trendy gyms you do all you can to get your heart rate up, like in HIIT workouts. Instead, Zone 2 cardio like walking on an incline is best along with stretching and mobility exercises. Adding in sprint interval training can help increase your VO2 (volume of oxygen) max, minding where you are at in your cycle. VO2 max is the maximum amount of oxygen your body can use during intense exercise. This is often used as a benchmark for athletic performance and cardiovascular health. An example would be five to six reps of 30 seconds at all-out effort sprint with a 60-second rest in between, during the follicular stage. More on cycle syncing later (see Chapter 10).

Lifting weights is going to be the best course of action. Muscle is an organ! It's an organ that keeps us strong, able to get up out of a chair, carry our babies, even move furniture around if needed. For me, it's so helpful when I am carrying all the Costo groceries in (remember, I have four children)!

Muscle is called the longevity organ. This is because muscle helps maintain optimal insulin sensitivity, allowing tissues to respond efficiently to glucose. Insulin resistance is a huge problem, and being metabolically flexible should be everyone's goal. A recent study showed that only 17.6% of Americans have optimal metabolic health.

What exactly does insulin resistance mean?

Remember the analogy to a song in Chapter 5? Have you ever listened to a song you love, and every time you hear it you get so excited and sing with your car windows down? Remember how after you hear it for the hundredth time, you don't get as enthusiastic about it? You have become resistant to it because you heard it so much.

This is what happens to cells over time when you consume too much refined sugar and carbohydrates. The cells become resistant to all of that sugar floating around in the body all the time. Extreme glucose spikes flood the body with insulin, and eventually the cells become resistant, and/or the pancreas gets burnt out from the extreme high blood sugars. Sounds exhausting, right? It is.

Why does this happen? In the U.S., everything is wrapped in a package of plastic (which alone is a hormone disruptor) and filled with refined sugar, carbohydrates, and seed oils. Over time, eating this way leads to insulin resistance. This can happen even if you are skinny! No one is safe. We all need to start paying attention to sugar (glucose) spikes.

Building muscle can help reverse insulin resistance and aid in preventing it too. I see patients who start lifting weights reduce their fasting insulin so quickly. It's truly impressive.

The Formula for Muscle Building in Perimenopause

1. Exercise: Prioritize strength training with progressive overload. Muscle growth starts with resistance training, which provides the necessary stimulus for muscles to adapt and grow stronger. Without it, even the best nutrition and supplementation won't yield significant muscle gains.
   - Focus on Progressive Overload: Gradually increase weights, reps, or intensity over time. This sends a clear signal to your body that it needs to prioritize muscle building.
   - Incorporate Compound Movements: Exercises like squats, deadlifts, bench presses, and rows work multiple muscle groups and promote overall strength.
   - Train Consistently: Aim for two to three sessions per week, allowing at least 48 hours of rest between sessions for muscle recovery. When not weightlifting, walking and stretching (mobility) exercises can be helpful.
2. Protein
   Protein is essential for muscle repair and growth. Think of it as the bricks for constructing new muscle tissue.

How Much Protein Do You Need?

- Aim for 1.2–2.0 grams of protein per kilogram of body weight daily. For example, if you weigh 70 kg (154 pounds), aim for 84–140 grams of protein per day.
- Older adults, including women in perimenopause, may benefit from slightly higher protein intake to counteract age-related muscle loss. Discuss with your integrative physician.
- Try for about 30 grams per meal!

Why Protein Is Crucial in Perimenopause:

- Muscle Preservation: Declining estrogen and testosterone reduce muscle protein synthesis. Higher protein helps maintain lean mass, which naturally declines with age.
- Metabolic Health: Muscle is metabolically active and helps regulate insulin sensitivity. Protein-rich diets help counter the rise in insulin resistance seen during perimenopause.
- Appetite & Satiety: Protein increases satiety hormones (like GLP-1 and peptide YY), helping manage weight and reduce cravings.
- Bone Health: Protein supports collagen production and works synergistically with calcium and vitamin D to maintain bone density, which is crucial since bone loss accelerates after estrogen declines.
- Sleep & Mood: Amino acids like tryptophan and glycine from protein are precursors to neurotransmitters (e.g., serotonin aids in feeling emotionally balanced. GABA helps calm and relax your brain, body, and nervous system), supporting mood stability and sleep quality.

Here are some ways to get 30 grams of protein:

Animal-Based Foods for 30 grams of Protein

Chicken: 4.5 oz (cooked, skinless)
Beef: 5 oz (cooked, lean cut)

Salmon: 5 oz (cooked)
Shrimp: 5 oz (cooked, ~20–25 medium shrimp)
Eggs: 5 large eggs
Greek Yogurt: 1.5 cups (plain, non-fat, ~300 g)
Cottage Cheese: 1 cup (low-fat, ~200 g)
Whey Protein: 1 scoop (30–35 g, depending on brand)

Check out my website for my favorite protein powders and protein-focused meal plans.

3. Amino Acids: Focus on leucine-rich foods or supplements to trigger muscle synthesis.
   - What are amino acids?
     - They are the individual units that make up protein. Of particular importance for muscle building are the branched-chain amino acids (BCAAs), especially leucine (helps muscles grow, repair, and stay strong).
   - Why Leucine Matters:
     - Leucine acts as a "trigger" for muscle protein synthesis. It signals your body to start building muscle after a meal or workout.
     - How Much Leucine: Aim for 2.5–3 grams per meal for optimal muscle synthesis.
     - Sources of Leucine: Eggs, chicken, beef, dairy
   - Why Essential Amino Acids (EAAs) Matter:
     - While leucine is key, all nine essential amino acids are required for muscle repair. Most complete proteins (e.g., meat, eggs, dairy) contain all EAAs. Vegetarians or vegans may need to combine foods (e.g., rice and beans) to get a full spectrum.

4. Creatine: Take 3–5 g daily to boost strength and recovery.
   - What Is Creatine?
     - Creatine is one of the most well-researched supplements for muscle growth and strength, and it becomes especially valuable during perimenopause. Creatine is a compound stored in muscle cells that provides quick bursts of energy during intense activity, like weightlifting. It also helps muscles recover and grow.
   - Why Creatine in Perimenopause?
     - Increases strength and power, allowing you to lift heavier weights and stimulate more muscle growth.
     - Improves muscle cell hydration, which can enhance protein synthesis.
     - Supports brain health and energy levels, which can be affected by hormonal shifts. Emerging research suggests that creatine may have a positive impact on cognitive performance, particularly in tasks requiring short-term memory and quick thinking. This is likely due to creatine's role in energy metabolism within the brain.
   - How to Use Creatine:
     - Dosage: Take 3–5 grams of creatine monohydrate daily. It's safe for prolonged use.
     - Timing: Creatine timing is flexible; you can take it before or after workouts or anytime during the day.
     - Hydration: Drink plenty of water, as creatine draws water into your muscles.
5. Whey Protein
   - Whey protein is a fast-digesting, complete protein source ideal for post-workout recovery. Studies show whey enhances muscle protein synthesis and supports lean mass preservation during weight loss.

6. PeptiStrong
   - What is PeptiStrong?
     - Derived from fava beans, PeptiStrong contains plant-based peptides shown to improve muscle recovery and reduce inflammation. It is suitable for individuals with dietary restrictions or plant-based preferences.
7. Recovery: Prioritize sleep, hydration, and active recovery.
   - Sleep supports growth hormone release and muscle protein synthesis. Without it, your body can't rebuild muscle after training.
   - Hydration maintains cellular function and muscle tissue elasticity, helping reduce soreness and optimizing performance.
   - Active recovery (gentle movement like walking or mobility work) improves circulation and helps clear metabolic byproducts, speeding up tissue repair.

Breast Cancer Concerns in Perimenopause: Evaluating High-Protein vs. Plant-Based Diets

During perimenopause, women experience fluctuations in estrogen and progesterone levels, which can influence breast tissue and potentially increase the risk of breast cancer. Elevated estrogen levels, particularly in estrogen receptor-positive (ER+) breast cancers, can promote tumor growth. However, high-protein diets can help stabilize insulin levels and reduce postprandial glucose spikes.

Studies have shown meals with a higher protein content led to less fluctuation in plasma glucose and insulin concentrations compared to meals lower in protein. This stabilization can be beneficial for metabolic health, particularly in perimenopausal women who may experience insulin resistance.

In addition, adequate protein intake is essential for maintaining muscle mass, especially during the perimenopausal phase when women may experience muscle loss due to hormonal changes. Research suggests that high-protein diets can support muscle preservation, which is crucial for overall health and metabolic function.

Despite these benefits, high-protein diets, particularly those rich in animal protein, have been linked to increased breast cancer risk. Some studies suggest that high intake of red and processed meats may elevate the risk of breast cancer due to the presence of hormones and carcinogenic compounds formed during cooking.

Plant-based foods are rich in phytoestrogens, which can mimic estrogen in the body and may help balance hormone levels. Plant-based diets can be high in antioxidants, vitamins, and minerals, which can combat oxidative stress and inflammation, two factors that contribute to cancer development. The anti-inflammatory properties of many plant foods may also play a role in reducing breast cancer risk.

When considering dietary patterns during perimenopause, it is essential to balance the benefits of high protein with the protective effects of plant-based foods. Both high-protein and plant-based diets have their respective benefits and risks concerning breast cancer in perimenopausal women. As research continues to evolve, women should consider their individual health needs and consult healthcare professionals when making dietary choices related to breast cancer risk.

Cultivate Perimenopause Supplementation

Perimenopause is a time of hormonal imbalance, with progesterone declining first and estrogen fluctuations that can lead to estrogen dominance. This imbalance creates symptoms like heavy periods, mood swings, bloating, and breast tenderness. To manage these, we need to:

1. Balance hormones like progesterone and DHEA.
2. Support estrogen detoxification (Phase 1, 2, and 3).
3. Address symptoms caused by estrogen dominance.
4. Reduce stress and support adrenal health.

Key Supplements for Perimenopause

Perimenopause calls for a selection of supplements that will work in your body's favor. Each plays their part in helping to harmonize your hormones. The following list summarizes each supplement's purpose and benefits.

1. Metabolic Balance
- Berberine
  Berberine can be particularly helpful during perimenopause due to its ability to:
  - Activate the AMPK Pathway (AMP-activated protein kinase pathway) a master energy sensor inside your cells. The AMPK Pathway enhances energy regulation, supports insulin sensitivity, reduces fat storage, promotes fat breakdown, and improves cellular energy and mitochondrial function.
  - Improve insulin sensitivity and reduce insulin resistance, helping manage weight and stabilize hormonal fluctuations.
  - Lower blood sugar, cholesterol, and triglycerides, reducing cardiovascular risks associated with perimenopause.
  - Decrease systemic inflammation and oxidative stress, easing symptoms like joint pain and fatigue.

- Inositol
  Inositol can help manage perimenopause symptoms by:
  - Enhancing insulin sensitivity, supporting better regulation of hormones affected by insulin resistance.
  - Supporting the regulation of neurotransmitters like serotonin, helping reduce anxiety and depression symptoms.
  - Calming the nervous system and helping to manage stress hormones, improving sleep quality.
  - Reducing the risk of insulin resistance, weight gain, and metabolic syndrome, which are common during perimenopause.
- Rhapontic Rhubarb Extract
  Rhapontic rhubarb extract (from *Rheum rhaponticum*) has been clinically shown to:
  - Alleviate common perimenopausal symptoms like hot flashes, night sweats, and mood swings.
  - Modulate estrogen receptors in a mild way that reduces estrogenic symptoms without increasing estrogen levels.
  - Help your body adjust to fluctuating estrogen levels.
    Think of rhapontic rhubarb as a calming guide for estrogen receptors..

2. Progesterone and Hormonal Balance (test, don't guess, hormone levels)
   - Vitex (Chasteberry):
     - Stimulates luteinizing hormone (LH) to promote natural progesterone production. Vitex acts on the hypothalamic-pituitary axis, particularly by modulating dopamine receptors, which in turn reduces prolactin levels. Prolactin is a hormone produced by the pituitary gland that plays a role in menstrual cycle regulation, ovulation, and breast development. Lower prolactin can normalize LH secretion, especially in women with prolactin-driven cycle irregularities.

- Helps regulate menstrual cycles, balance mood, and reduce breast tenderness.
- Bioidentical Progesterone Cream or capsules under physician supervision:
  - Directly supplements progesterone, offsetting estrogen dominance.
  - Useful for calming mood, promoting sleep, and regulating periods.

3. DHEA and Adrenal Support
- DHEA Supplementation:
  - Restores declining DHEA levels, which support libido, mood, and overall hormone balance.
  - Consult a healthcare provider to avoid excess, which can lead to androgenic effects like acne or facial hair growth. Test levels, don't guess.
- Adaptogens (e.g., Ashwagandha, Rhodiola Rosea):
  - Reduce stress and cortisol production, sparing pregnenolone for sex hormone synthesis.
  - Support energy levels and resilience during hormonal fluctuations.

A Comprehensive Plan for Perimenopause

Category	Supplement	Purpose
Hormonal Balance	Vitex, Bioidentical Progesterone Cream	Boost progesterone, regulate cycles
Estrogen Detox	Calcium D-Glucarate, Milk Thistle, NAC	Support liver detox and estrogen removal
Hot Flashes/Mood Swings	Rhapontic Rhubarb Extract	Reduce vasomotor symptoms, stabilize mood
Stress & Energy	Ashwagandha, Rhodiola Rosea, DHEA	Support adrenal health, reduce cortisol
Bone & Overall Health	Calcium, Vitamin D3 + K2, Magnesium	Maintain bone density and cardiovascular health
Anti-Inflammatory Support	Omega-3 Fatty Acids	Reduce inflammation, improve mood
Metabolism	Inositol, Berberine	Balance glucose to insulin, promotes insulin sensitivity

When buying supplements, make sure you are ordering them from a trusted source. The internet can have supplements that are contaminated with heavy metals or are adulterated—not what they say they are! This can clog your liver instead of helping it. Check out my resources on where to purchase supplements.

Cultivate a Smart Nutrition Plan to Address Hormonal Shifts

Nutrition that supports hormone balance is imperative during perimenopause. A tailored nutrition plan will set you up for success on this journey. In the following pages, you will learn more about the foods and nutrients that will significantly support your overall health.

When it comes to nutrition, your objectives are to focus on healthy fats and optimal protein.

Healthy Fats

These fats are stable, nutrient-dense, and beneficial for overall health:

- Butter:
  - Is rich in fat-soluble vitamins (A, D, E, K).
  - Contains conjugated linoleic acid (CLA), which may support metabolism and heart health.
  - Is high in saturated fats, making it heat-stable for cooking.
- Tallow (beef fat):
  - Is an excellent source of saturated and monounsaturated fats.
  - Has a high smoke point, making it ideal for frying and baking.
  - Contains fat-soluble vitamins and supports hormone production.
- Lard (pork fat):
  - Is rich in monounsaturated fats (like olive oil).
  - Is high in vitamin D, especially from pastured pigs.
  - Is versatile for cooking due to its mild flavor and stability.
- Olive Oil (extra virgin):
  - Is rich in heart-healthy monounsaturated fats and antioxidants.

- Has anti-inflammatory properties, linked to reduced risk of chronic diseases.
- Has a moderate smoke point, best used for low-to-medium heat or raw applications like salads.
- Avocado Oil:
  - Is high in monounsaturated fats and vitamin E.
  - Has a neutral flavor and high smoke point that make it multipurpose—perfect for frying or other cooking methods
  - Supports skin health and reduces inflammation.

Why Seed Oils Are Problematic

Seed oils (such as soybean, canola, corn, sunflower, and safflower oil) are unstable, highly processed, and prone to oxidation. Here's why:

- High in Omega-6 Fatty Acids:
  - Seed oils are rich in omega-6 fats, which can cause inflammation when consumed in excess relative to omega-3s.
  - This imbalance is linked to chronic diseases like heart disease, obesity, and autoimmune disorders.
- Easily Oxidized:
  - Seed oils are polyunsaturated, making them chemically unstable. When exposed to heat, light, or oxygen, they oxidize, forming harmful free radicals.
  - Oxidation can damage cells, promote inflammation, and contribute to aging and disease.
- Heavily Processed:
  - Seed oils undergo industrial extraction processes using high heat and chemical solvents, which degrade their quality.
  - These processes also introduce harmful byproducts like trans fats.
- Anti-Nutrient Effects:
  - Excess omega-6 fats can interfere with the body's ability to use omega-3s effectively, impairing brain function, immunity, and heart health.

- Linked to Health Issues:
    - Chronic inflammation from oxidized seed oils is associated with metabolic syndrome, cancer, and neurodegenerative diseases.

Stick to stable, natural fats like butter, tallow, lard, olive oil, and avocado oil. These fats are nutrient-rich, heat-stable, and far less prone to oxidation than seed oils, making them a healthier choice for cooking and overall health. Avoid seed oils due to their instability, inflammatory effects, and poor nutrient profile.

Why You Should Avoid Seed Oils

Seed oils, particularly those high in polyunsaturated fatty acids (PUFAs), have garnered criticism for their potential health risks, primarily due to their susceptibility to oxidation. When seed oils are exposed to heat, light, or air, they can undergo oxidative degradation, leading to the formation of harmful compounds that may negatively impact health. This oxidation process can produce free radicals and other reactive oxygen species, which are known to contribute to inflammation and various chronic diseases, including cardiovascular disease and cancer. We love tallow and butter in our kitchen!

ANIMAL-BASED PROTEINS

These provide complete proteins, containing all nine essential amino acids that your body needs.

- Eggs:
    - Are rich in high-quality protein, choline (important for brain health), and healthy fats.

- Contain antioxidants like lutein and zeaxanthin, which are both natural pigments that safeguard your eyes and help maintain eye health.
- Beef (grass-fed, if possible):
  - Is an excellent source of iron, zinc, and B vitamins.
  - Is rich in complete proteins and healthy fats, especially from grass-fed sources.
- Poultry (chicken, turkey):
  - Are lean protein options that are versatile and widely available.
  - Dark meat provides more fat and iron, while white meat is leaner.
- Fish (salmon, sardines, mackerel, cod):
  - Is high in omega-3 fatty acids, especially fatty fish like salmon and sardines.
  - Is rich in iodine, selenium, and vitamin D, supporting thyroid and brain health.
- Lamb:
  - Is rich in heme iron, conjugated linoleic acid (CLA), and complete protein.
  - Is typically grass-fed, making it a good source of omega-3s.
- Pork (pastured or heritage-raised):
  - Contains complete protein and nutrients like thiamine, selenium, and zinc.
  - Avoid highly processed options like bacon or sausage unless they are minimally processed. Look for nitrate/nitrite-free varieties.

Dairy-Based Proteins (if tolerated)

- Greek Yogurt:
  - Is high in protein and probiotics, supporting gut health.
  - Choose plain, full-fat options to avoid added sugars.

- Cheese:
  - Is nutrient-dense and high in calcium, protein, and healthy fats.
  - Hard cheeses (like Parmesan) are particularly high in protein.
- Cottage Cheese:
  - Is a lean protein source rich in casein, which digests slowly and helps with muscle repair.

Prioritize Quality: Grass-fed, pasture-raised, or wild-caught options are often higher in nutrients and healthier fats. Get to know your local farmers, visit their farms, and buy from them.

Best Artificial Sweeteners

When choosing artificial or natural sugar alternatives, prioritize those with minimal impact on blood sugar and fewer side effects:

- Stevia:
  - Pros: Plant-based, zero calories, and does not spike blood sugar.
  - Cons: Some find it has a slight bitter aftertaste.
  - Best Use: Sweetening drinks, baking (combined with other sweeteners to offset the aftertaste).
- Monk Fruit:
  - Pros: Derived from a fruit, with zero calories, no glycemic impact, and a milder taste than stevia.
  - Cons: Often blended with other sweeteners; ensure purity when purchasing. Many brands are cut with erythritol.
  - Best Use: Great for beverages, desserts, and sauces.
- Allulose:
  - Pros: A rare sugar with only 1/10th the calories of regular sugar and no significant impact on blood sugar or insulin.
  - Cons: Consuming large amounts may cause digestive discomfort for some.
  - Best Use: Perfect for baking, as it behaves like sugar in recipes.

Best-in-Class Vegetables (Low Oxalate, Low Phytic Acid)

Choose nutrient-dense, low-anti-nutrient vegetables that are easier on digestion and promote overall health.

Oxalates and phytic acid can interfere with mineral absorption—like calcium, iron, and zinc—and may contribute to kidney stones, anemia, or gut irritation in sensitive individuals.

This is especially important during perimenopause, when declining estrogen increases the risk of bone loss, iron deficiency, and digestive sensitivity.

Remember how vital it is to choose vegetables that support nutrient absorption and hormonal balance.

- Broccoli:
    - Is low in oxalates and phytic acid.
    - Is rich in vitamin C, K, and fiber.
    - Supports detoxification and gut health.
- Brussels Sprouts:
    - Are low in oxalates and moderate in phytic acid.
    - Are high in fiber, vitamin K, and glucosinolates.
    - Support estrogen metabolism and liver detox pathways.
- Green Beans:
    - Are low in oxalates and high in fiber.
    - Provide potassium and folate.
    - Are gentle on digestion compared to other legumes.
- Zucchini:
    - Is low in oxalates.
    - Is easy to digest.
    - Is rich in antioxidants and hydration.
- Cauliflower:
    - Is low in oxalates.
    - Is packed with vitamin C, fiber, and choline.
- Cabbage:
    - Is low in anti-nutrients.
    - Is supportive of gut health.
    - Its high sulfur content aids detox.

- Cucumber:
  - Is hydrating.
  - Is low in anti-nutrients.
  - Is mild on the stomach.

TOP-SHELF FRUITS (FOCUS ON BERRIES)

Berries are nutrient-dense, low in sugar, and high in antioxidants, making them ideal for most diets.

- Blueberries:
  - Are high in antioxidants like anthocyanins (natural plant pigments).
  - Support brain and heart health.
  - Have a low glycemic index.
- Raspberries:
  - Are rich in fiber, vitamin C, and antioxidants.
  - Are excellent for blood sugar control and gut health.
- Strawberries:
  - Are high in vitamin C and manganese.
  - Have a low sugar content.
- Blackberries:
  - Are loaded with fiber, vitamin K, and antioxidants.
- Cranberries (unsweetened):
  - Are great for urinary tract health.
  - Are rich in polyphenols.

EXPLORING CARNIVORE AND ANIMAL-BASED DIETS

Carnivore and animal-based diets focus on nutrient-dense animal products and often limit plant foods. Here's how they align with perimenopause:

- Core Principles:
  - Carnivore: Exclusively animal products (meat, organs, fish, eggs, animal fats, and sometimes dairy).

- Animal-Based: Emphasizes animal products but allows some low-toxin plant foods like fruit, honey, and low-oxalate vegetables.
- Benefits:
  - Nutrient density: High in bioavailable vitamins (A, D, B12, K2) and minerals like heme iron and zinc.
  - Lower anti-nutrients: Eliminate oxalates, lectins, and phytic acid found in plant foods that can impair nutrient absorption.
  - Hormonal support: Rich in cholesterol and healthy fats, crucial for hormone synthesis.

> Pay careful attention, then, to how you walk,
> not as unwise people but as wise.
>
> —Ephesians 5:15 (CSB)

Perimenopause is a season of transition, but it's also a powerful invitation to walk wisely—to be intentional with how you care for your body. This verse reminds us to live with discernment, not on autopilot.

What you put in your body can either create inflammation or heal your body. The foods you eat, the workouts you choose, and the way you manage rest and stress all shape how your body navigates this transition.

Wisdom in this season means tuning in to what your body truly needs, not just following what worked in your 20s. You are not out of control—you are in a position of stewardship. Walk wisely. Choose healing.

Peptides in Perimenopause

What role do peptides play in supporting women through perimenopause? As hormones begin to shift and symptoms emerge—from fatigue and weight gain to poor recovery and cognitive fog—could targeted peptides offer a science-backed way to support hormone signaling, tissue repair, and overall vitality during this transition?

Peptides and Their Role in Perimenopause

Peptides are short chains of amino acids that act as signaling molecules in the body, helping regulate various processes like inflammation, tissue repair, and metabolism. During perimenopause, when hormonal fluctuations can lead to systemic imbalances, peptides can play a supportive role in alleviating symptoms. These promote overall well-being and address underlying issues such as inflammation, metabolism, and tissue repair.

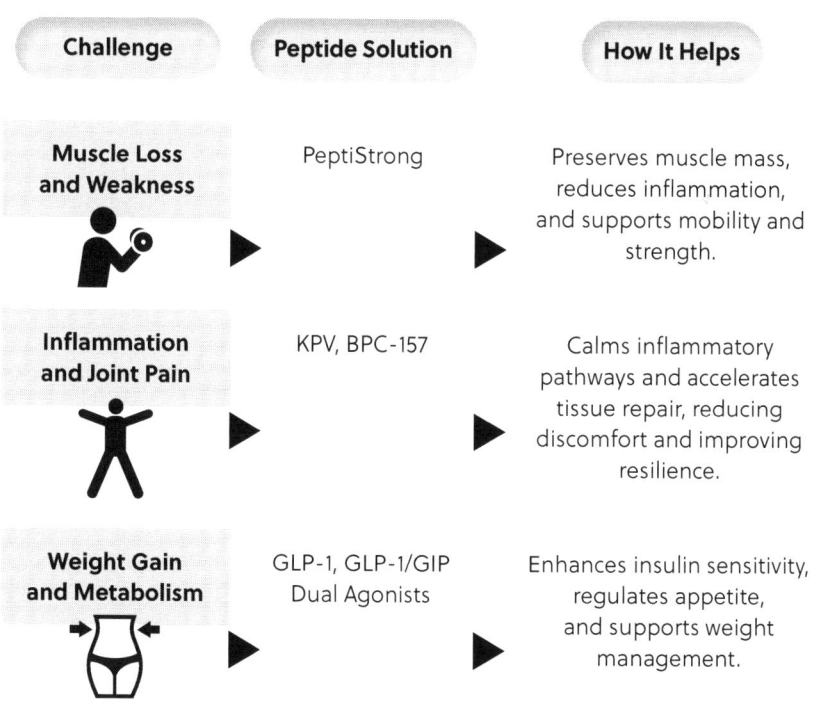

Key Peptides and Their Potential Benefits During Perimenopause

Challenge	Peptide Solution	How It Helps
Muscle Loss and Weakness	PeptiStrong	Preserves muscle mass, reduces inflammation, and supports mobility and strength.
Inflammation and Joint Pain	KPV, BPC-157	Calms inflammatory pathways and accelerates tissue repair, reducing discomfort and improving resilience.
Weight Gain and Metabolism	GLP-1, GLP-1/GIP Dual Agonists	Enhances insulin sensitivity, regulates appetite, and supports weight management.

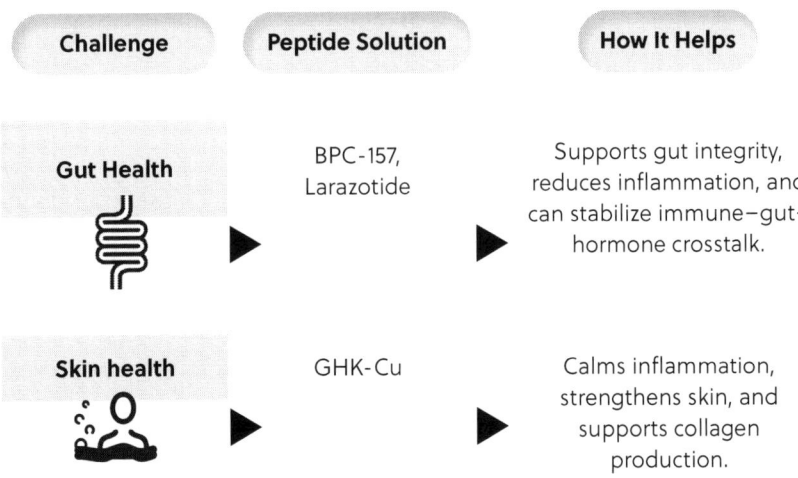

For more information, check out the resources section.

> The Lord will always lead you, stratify you in a parched land and strengthen your bones, you will be like a watered garden and like a spring whose water never runs dry.
>
> —Isaiah 58:11 (CSB)

Remember Ada? She took the steps to get her health back by getting proper rest, increasing protein and healthy fats, and going back to weight training. With the help of supplements and a luteal phase progesterone and oral DHEA, she was able get her hormones balanced again while in the depths of perimenopause. It can be done! Our bodies are very resilient.

Many women get frustrated at how they feel and think it's not normal. It happens all the time, but your body is able to recover if you have the correct tools. Let the Lord lead you in this adventure, and use wisdom in your health journey.

Chapter Key Takeaways:

- Hormonal shifts during perimenopause impact muscle repair, muscle loss, and stress levels
- Exercise (lifting weights), nutrition, and supplementation are integral to optimizing your hormone balance
- Peptides can provide symptom relief and help address inflammation, tissue repair, and metabolism

Part 3:
Spirit

This part might be difficult for some of you to read. It might feel uncomfortable. You may even feel convicted—and that's okay. But please know this: there is no condemnation here. I'm going to share some deeply personal stories, so you know you're not alone. We're walking through this together, with grace and truth, not shame.

Over the last decade, it has been glaringly obvious that our health is not just tied to our physical body, but to our spiritual body as well. I have seen this so many times at my office when dealing with patients that it is undeniable. Strongholds, hexes, curses, and bloodline factors—all can come into play.

We can also be easily deceived by external forces in the world (I was), impacting our relationship with Christ. The thing is that, as Christians, we are not always told about spiritual warfare, even though the Bible discusses it. I've spoken with several pastors who've shared that they try to be cautious about discussing heavier topics—like spiritual warfare—because they don't want to overwhelm or scare people off when they attend church.

> For our struggle is not against flesh and blood,
> but against the rulers, against the authorities, against the powers of this dark world, and against the spiritual forces of evil in the heavenly realms.
>
> —Ephesians 6:12 (NIV)

It had to be so obvious to me that I couldn't deny it. As a scientist and a physician, I needed proof. There is nothing like experiencing spiritual warfare yourself.

The real challenge for those of us who grasp the reality of spiritual warfare isn't avoiding discomfort—it's awakening awareness. Our goal isn't to frighten people; it's to help them recognize what they're already experiencing, often without a name for it. Because once someone sees the battle for what it is, they can finally begin to fight back: not in fear, but in the freedom and authority that comes with walking in step with Jesus.

I believe that women are especially targeted by the enemy during perimenopause. In this season of physical and emotional vulnerability, we can also be more prone to the pull of the flesh and the temptation to rely on ourselves instead of God's sustaining grace. Think back to friends who got divorced, dove into New Age stuff ("Oh hey, I'm doing yoga teacher training!"), ran a marathon (we discussed why this can push you over the hormonal cliff), went to Taylor Swift concerts (no judgment, but we need awareness about secular music—more on that later), or got started on antidepressants, all of which can leave us more vulnerable to the enemy's schemes.

> Be alert and of sober mind.
> Your enemy the devil prowls around like
> a roaring lion looking for someone to devour.
>
> —1 Peter 5:8 (NIV)

Ann sat across from me at my office desk. She was doing really well with her health, her hormones were balanced, and her menstrual cycle was more regular. Ann was eating healthy, hitting her protein goals.

"It's odd," she said. "A few times a month, I will be driving home and suddenly be in the parking lot of McDonald's drinking a Coke and eating fries. I don't know how it happens. It's almost like I am in a trance."

I sat back in my chair, and told her, "This is definitely spiritual. We need to pray over this, rebuke the spirit of gluttony, and deal with any pride that keeps you from trusting God."

Has this happened to you? Do you feel like you are doing so well and then self-sabotage for no reason? The Lord didn't create us to numb our feelings via food addiction. This can be spiritual warfare. We also are at constant battle with sin, acting out our own fallen nature—the flesh, pulling us toward disobedience.

> For the desires of the flesh are against the Spirit,
> and the desires of the Spirit are against the flesh,
> for these are opposed to each other,
> to keep you from doing the things you want to do.
>
> —Galatians 5:17 ESV

I am praying for you reading this book right now. Praying that God gives you ears to listen and eyes to see, so you can experience real freedom in your health and healing. I believe you are not here by accident—He has chosen you. Before the foundation of the world, He knew your name, your story, and this very moment.

Even in the tough parts of your health journey, His purpose remains steady. You've been set apart—not because of anything you've done, but because of His grace.

CHAPTER 7

Cleanse: Release to Restore

Heal the sick, bring the dead back to life, heal those who suffer from dreaded skin diseases, and drive out demons. You have received without paying, so give without being paid.

—Matthew 10:8 (GNT)

If we're called to bring healing, we must first remove what is toxic. The music we listen to, the books we read, and the people we welcome into close relationship can either speak life into us or slowly drain it away.

This chapter is an invitation to take inventory—to cleanse what doesn't align with truth and make space for what brings peace, clarity, and Christ-centered restoration.

Surround Yourself with Good Things

On Music: Fill Your Ears with What Feeds Your Soul

Have you ever noticed the lyrics you are singing and what they actually mean? The songs that your children are listening to, learning, and unintentionally memorizing?

A few years ago, I began listening to Christian music all the time. I play it in the car, at the gym, and in the house. It has been life changing. Before, I was still listening mostly to alternative rock. Some of the bands were Christian, but most were not. Why would I be listening to something that wouldn't fill my mind and heart with more of sweet Jesus?

The best thing about playing Christian music is that my kids will just start singing along. It's amazing. I love to blast some tunes and sing at the top of my lungs; I will also start crying if the lyrics move me. It's great. Cleanse what you hear in your home, in your car, and while you work out. Make the switch for two months and notice what you discover. Also, the concerts are amazing. Bring your children!

Here Are a Few of My Favorite Christian Bands

Here are a Few of My Favorite Christian Bands: Forrest Frank, Journey Worship Co, Lauren Daigle, Mercy Me, Love & the Outcome, Hulvey, Anne Wilson, and For King and Country, just to name a few!

ON BOOKS: FEEDING THE MIND TO FUEL THE MISSION

What about books? Obviously, I am a self-proclaimed nerd. I devour scientific books, books on integrative medicine, and of course I spend many hours reading medical case studies. My bookshelves are lined with pages that stretch my thinking, deepen my practice, and inspire me to serve better.

What has also been life changing during perimenopause is reading faith-based books and recommending them to friends so we can talk about them together. The conversations that followed brought encouragement, wisdom, and deeper connection. Even better? Join or start a Christ-centered book club. The best relationships I have formed have been at my friend's book club. Attendance was a non-negotiable, and we would stay late, laughing, crying, and praying.

What books are you reading? Are they building you up or breaking you down? Just like food can either cause inflammation or bring healing to the body, the content we consume—what we read, watch, and fill our minds with—can either nourish our spirit or slowly wear it down.

My son had an experience in public school that truly opened our eyes. In fourth grade, his teacher read a book to the entire class about a young child who was transgender. When he came home and told us, he was clearly uncomfortable. He felt it wasn't appropriate to share something so complex with such young, impressionable students.

Long story short—he bravely spoke up at a school board meeting, and as a result, new policies were put in place to protect students. But after that, things changed for him. He was treated differently at school by the teachers and staff. It was hard.

Still, that moment of courage led us down a new path—one that brought us to homeschooling and alternative educational resources that have truly been a blessing for him and for our whole family.

Check out my favorite books linked in the resources.

As iron sharpens iron, so one person sharpens another.

—Proverbs 27:17 (NIV)

On Friendship: Sanctified Together

As women, we don't just *crave* connection—we're *created* for it. Godly friendship isn't about surface-level support; it's about soul-deep sanctification. Real fellowship means loving each other enough to speak truth—not to shame, but to sharpen.

This isn't a call-out culture—it's a call-up culture.

Through grace-filled honesty, we help one another grow, heal, and become more like Christ. That's the beauty of Spirit-led sisterhood.

We were meant to find fellowship. Not just friends that talk about kids' sports or the weather, but friends you get deep with. You share your worst fears, and they pray over you and tell you that God's in control. You leave feeling lighter and with hope. However, the enemy will find ways and give you excuses for you not to have those types of friendships.

As an adult, you will need to make choices about the friendships that you will maintain. Keep this in mind: Will you choose friends who will draw you closer to the kingdom or who will push you away? The other thing to consider is the effect this will have on your children and their children.

You need to pray, ask, and knock:

> Ask and it will be given to you; seek and you will find;
> knock and the door will be opened to you.
>
> —Matthew 7:7 (NIV)

You've probably heard the saying, often attributed to motivational speaker Jim Rohn, that "you are the average of the five people you spend the most time with." I like to take that one step further—and think of it through the lens of gut health.

> Whoever walks with the wise becomes wise,
> but the companion of fools will suffer harm.
>
> —Proverbs 13:20 ESV

Emerging research shows that the people we spend the most time with—family, close friends, even roommates—often share more than just values or habits. We actually share parts of our microbiomes. Through shared environments, frequent close contact, and similar diets, our gut bacteria begin to look more alike. And since the gut is deeply connected to our mood, cognition, and overall well-being, the company we keep may be shaping us in more ways than we realize.

Do we want to become more like the world (sin), or more like Jesus? What do you want your spiritual microbiome to look like?

On Emotions: Letting Go of Anger Before It Grips You

> In your anger do not sin:
> Do not let the sun go down while you are still angry,
> and do not give the devil a foothold.
>
> —Ephesians 4:26–27 (NIV)

I used to choose anger, because I am a sinner. And while there is such a thing as righteous anger, that's not the same as being short-tempered or perpetually irritated. We all fall into moods, but unchecked anger opens a door to sin. Do we even need anger? As Dallas Willard once said, "Anything done in anger can be done better without it."

Choose to be grateful in every situation, and you will not only feel joy; you will shine joy. Don't fake it, either. Write down three things you are grateful for every day and talk about it with your family at dinner. Share gratitude in evening prayers. Studies show that gratitude can broaden thinking, attention, and build personal resources that can help foster physical health and resilience.

On Film and TV Shows: Nourish Mind, Body, Spirit with Uplifting Media

Psychology tells us what many of us already feel instinctively: what we watch matters. Whether it's a suspense-filled Netflix series or a chilling horror film, consuming fear-based or emotionally disturbing media leaves a mark on the brain.

Research shows that these forms of entertainment can increase anxiety, disrupt brain connectivity, and even impair cognitive performance. More importantly, the effects often linger long after the screen goes dark, subtly reshaping how our brains process emotion and stress. The media we consume becomes part of our mental and emotional diet—so let's choose wisely.

BDNF (Brain-Derived Neurotrophic Factor) is a protein that supports the growth, survival, and maintenance of neurons in the brain. It plays a critical role in neuroplasticity, learning, memory, and overall brain health, and its levels can be boosted through exercise, healthy diets, and certain supplements.

High cortisol levels during perimenopause can suppress progesterone production because the body prioritizes cortisol production over progesterone, as both rely on the same precursor, pregnenolone. See why this is a problem? Why are we still watching the news?

My parents sometimes watch CSI right before bed. Please don't do this too! I used to watch movies that had violence in them. Now, I refuse to—it's not worth it. Why affect my body/brain negatively and potentially open up doors to the demonic spiritual world?

Scripture says:

> Finally, brothers and sisters, whatever is true, whatever is noble, whatever is right, whatever is pure, whatever is lovely, whatever is admirable—if anything is excellent or praiseworthy—think about such things.
>
> —Philippians 4:8 (NIV)

Why are we watching things that don't do this? Listening to music that has corrupting lyrics? When it comes to healing and deliverance, we need to want the deliverer, not the deliverance. We need to seek Jesus first.

> Walk with the wise and become wise;
> associate with fools and get in trouble.
> —Proverbs 13:20 (NLT)

Get rid of toxicity, negativity, and bad TV shows that cue the sympathetic nervous system's fight-or-flight response. Toxicity and negativity in our environment, including exposure to distressing shows, can perpetuate a state of chronic stress. This keeps the body operating in the sympathetic fight-or-flight mode, which is great when meant for short-term survival but becomes harmful when prolonged. Chronic activation of this stress response can lead to issues like high blood pressure, weakened immunity, and mental health challenges such as anxiety and depression.

Adverse Childhood Experiences (ACEs) further compound this issue. ACEs are potentially traumatic events that occur during childhood, such as abuse, neglect, loss of a parent, or growing up in a household with mental health or substance use problems. Research shows that ACEs can have long-term effects on health, increasing the risk of chronic diseases like heart disease, diabetes, and depression. For example, individuals with an ACE score of four or more are significantly more likely to experience mental health challenges and chronic illnesses.

ACEs and Perimenopause

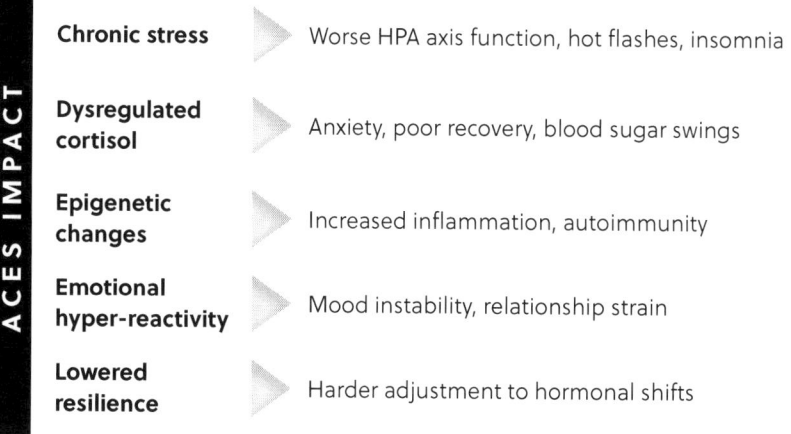

ACEs Impact		Result in Perimenopause
Chronic stress	→	Worse HPA axis function, hot flashes, insomnia
Dysregulated cortisol	→	Anxiety, poor recovery, blood sugar swings
Epigenetic changes	→	Increased inflammation, autoimmunity
Emotional hyper-reactivity	→	Mood instability, relationship strain
Lowered resilience	→	Harder adjustment to hormonal shifts

> Do not be misled: Bad company
> corrupts good character.
>
> —1 Corinthians 15:33 (NIV)

Cleanse Your Environment of Toxicity and Negativity

Detox Your Inputs – Spiritually and Mentally

Take a moment to reflect on what you're feeding your soul through media. Are the TV shows, social media feeds, or podcasts you engage with lifting you up—or pulling you down? If it stirs anxiety, comparison, or a sense of unrest, it might be time to lovingly let it go. Replace it with content that brings you closer to truth, wisdom, and peace—things that nourish your spirit and align with your walk with God. With God's help, you can be mindful of what you take in. As you rely on His strength, your faith and discernment will grow.

Protect Your Nervous System Peace

Living in constant fight-or-flight mode is like trying to rest while the fire alarm blares. Toxic environments and negative messaging overstimulate your sympathetic nervous system, elevating cortisol, disrupting digestion, impairing sleep, and eroding mental clarity. God designed your body for peace, not panic. Choose stillness. Choose input that calms, not chaos.

> When you feel spiritually attacked, overwhelmed, or exposed to darkness—whether through harsh words, spiritual opposition, or fear—pray not from panic, but from confidence in Christ's finished work. These prayers are rooted in God's Word and His sovereign protection.

> **A prayer for protection:**
>
> Lord, I trust in Your power and covering. Let no scheme of the enemy prevail. Guard me and my family, and let Your truth be my shield. Thank you that in Christ, I am secure.

> You, dear children, are from God and have overcome them, because the one who is in you is greater than the one who is in the world.
>
> —1 John 4:4 (NIV)

He who is in you is greater than the world. Do not focus on worldly things but instead give your attention to things that glorify God, and you will find peace. Cleanse your home, your Netflix account (better yet, check out Pureflix), and your activities. Test it with the Holy Spirit, the Bible, and prayer.

This might not seem easy, but it is—especially if you already tossed your perfume and stopped eating gluten!

When it comes to the cleansing process, or sanctification, we need to make sure we aren't comparing ourselves to others. Your chapter one is different from my chapter eight. I used to drink Diet Pepsi and stopped reading my Bible regularly in residency because I was busy becoming a doctor.

Sometimes you can drift off path so slowly that you don't notice you aren't still steered toward Jesus. We all have to start somewhere, but know this, what you have done in the past, He uses for good. It will become your testimony.

Chapter Key Takeaways:

- Feed your mind, body, and soul with faith-based books and music
- Be mindful of the friendships you keep: Are they uplifting and pulling you closer to the Kingdom of God?
- Cleanse your content consumption: Let go of toxic media and replace with content that brings peace

CHAPTER 8

CONNECT TO JESUS

I was first introduced to yoga during medical school. Later, during my fellowship in integrative medicine, I pursued it more and enrolled in teacher training. At the time, I even envisioned opening a yoga studio as part of my integrative health practice.

But somewhere along the way, I was replacing sacred time reading my Bible with spiritual yoga practices that didn't point me to Jesus. I found myself reading mantras instead of Scripture, seeking answers in reiki sessions instead of through prayer. Meditation became about emptying my mind—when what I truly needed was to fill it with God's truth.

In yoga, you're taught to let go, to clear your thoughts. But an empty mind without spiritual discernment is vulnerable. The enemy thrives in emptiness. What I needed was not just peace—but *His* presence.

> When an unclean spirit comes out of a person,
> it roams through waterless places looking for rest but doesn't find any. Then it says, "I'll go back to my house that I came from."
> Returning, it finds the house vacant, swept, and put in order.
> Then it goes and brings with it seven other spirits more evil than itself, and they enter and settle down there.
> As a result, that person's last condition is worse than the first.
> That's how it will also be with this evil generation.
>
> —Matthew 12:43–45 (CSB)

I've lived it.

I once embraced the self-help movement—the "I am enough" affirmations, the endless striving for self-empowerment. But instead of peace, it left me feeling emptier. More lost.

Before my youngest son was born, I experienced a miscarriage. I turned to my faith during that heartbreak, but true peace still eluded me. Looking back, I believe it was because I was still entangled in the mindset of the New Age. I hadn't fully surrendered.

During my integrative medicine fellowship, we were offered an optional drum circle. It seemed harmless. I participated, and during that time, I brought up my miscarriage. It felt like healing—but not the kind that comes from God. It was fleeting, incomplete, and left a deeper ache.

Years ago, when Apple changed their iPhone chargers, we all realized quickly that the wrong plug simply wouldn't work. It's the same with the spiritual life. You can try all the "universal" outlets—New Age practices, self-help books, yoga, secular music, even complete immersion in work or wellness—but if you're not plugged into Jesus, you're not getting true power or peace.

And I know, because I was deep in it. I was a certified yoga instructor. I owned a yoga studio that was attached to my integrative medicine clinic. I thought I was blending the best of both worlds.

But what I found was this: the more I took my eyes off Jesus, the more disconnected I became—from God, from truth, from real healing.

By His grace, I found my way back. And on the other side of surrender, I discovered a deeper relationship with God—and health, joy, and peace that undoubtedly lasted.

New Age / Syncretistic Language to Watch For

These words and phrases are often used to shift focus away from God toward self, vague "energy," or universal forces:

Universal / Energy Language

- The Universe (e.g., "Trust the Universe")
- Universal consciousness
- Vibrations / Raise your vibration
- Energy healing
- Alignment (without reference to God)
- Manifest / Manifestation
- Divine energy
- Frequencies

Self-Directed Empowerment

- You are enough
- You are your own healer
- Your higher self
- Trust yourself
- Look within
- Everything you need is already inside you
- Follow your truth
- You are limitless

Mystical / Occult Terms

- Third eye
- Awakening / Ascension
- Sacred geometry
- Spirit guides
- Channeling
- Crystal healing
- Past lives / karma
- Akashic records

Eastern Religious Concepts
(When Syncretized)

- Namaste (when used beyond cultural courtesy to imply divine self-worship)
- Prana / life force
- Kundalini
- Chakras
- Non-duality
- Oneness (as in dissolving individual identity)

If I keep my eyes on God, I won't trip over my own healer.

—Psalm 25:15 (MSG)

Yoga: Deceitful Peace and Hidden Darkness

The view of yoga as "demonic" is rooted in concerns about idolatry, cultural appropriation, and the perceived spiritual risks associated with its practice.

Yoga has its origins in ancient India, where it was practiced as a means of spiritual growth and connection with the divine. The term "yoga" itself means "to yoke" or "to unite," and it encompasses various paths, including bhakti yoga (the path of devotion), jnana yoga (the path of knowledge), and karma yoga (the path of selfless action). Each of these paths can involve practices that are considered devotional in nature.

Some yoga postures are explicitly named after Hindu deities or are associated with specific mythological stories. For instance, the "Goddess Pose" (*Utkata Konasana*) and "Warrior Pose" (*Virabhadrasana*) are named after divine figures and warriors in Hindu mythology. These positions can be seen as forms of homage or respect to these deities, embodying their qualities and energies during practice.

One of the most well-known sequences in yoga, *Surya Namaskar*, is traditionally performed as a form of worship to the sun god, *Surya*. Each posture in this sequence can be viewed as a salutation to the sun, expressing gratitude and reverence. This practice illustrates how yoga can serve as a spiritual ritual, connecting practitioners to the divine through physical movement.

This is a slippery slope to participate in as a Christian. Let me tell you from personal experience, it does open spiritual doors to the demonic.

> And no wonder! For Satan disguises himself as an angel of light.
>
> —2 Corinthians 11:14 (CSB)

I say this not as an outsider, but as someone who once stood on the inside. I was a yoga teacher, running my own studio. I led classes. And I was convinced I was doing something good.

Looking back, I see how yoga targets women, especially those in vulnerable seasons like perimenopause. It offers community, emotional relief, and empowerment—but subtly redirects your focus. The worship shifts away from Christ and toward the "universe," mantras, energy, and self.

It's packaged as healing. But it leads us to rely on practices that unlock spiritual doors not meant to be opened. If something stirs in you as you read this, take it seriously. Ask God for discernment. Step away. And if you've wandered off course, repent and return to reading the Bible. Jesus is always ready to welcome you home—with truth, not illusion.

What are the alternatives? You can stretch and do mobility workouts without practicing yoga. Go for a walk in nature or follow a non-yoga mobility work out. Gentle movement can calm the mind, balance the nervous system, and increase endorphins.

- Things that help with stress: prayer, being in nature, breath work, talking with trusted friends and family, adaptogen supplements, reading the Bible.
- Things that don't help: alcohol, gossip, New Age practices, hours on social media, Netflix binges.

Stress Reduction with Meditation and Breathwork: Natural Support for Perimenopause

Let's talk about stress.

Did you know that stress doesn't just make you feel older—it actually ages you on a cellular level? It shortens your telomeres, those tiny caps on the ends of your DNA that naturally get shorter as we age.

Telomere length has become the latest obsession in the biohacking world. You'll hear people brag, "My telomeres are the same as a 17-year-old's!" (Usually, men with no children ... go figure.)

Jokes aside—this matters. Chronically elevated cortisol (your main stress hormone) is linked to nearly every chronic illness, including cancer. And if that doesn't get your attention, consider this: high cortisol also disrupts your hormones, packs on stubborn weight, and can even cause hair thinning. Now are you listening?

> She is clothed with strength and dignity;
> she can laugh at the days to come.
>
> —Proverbs 31:25 (NIV)

This passage describes the noble, virtuous woman whose trust is in the Lord. These words remind me that even in uncertain times, we can face each day with courage and peace. The truth is, we can't eliminate stress, but by God's grace, we can choose how we respond.

What are some things that help with stress resilience?

Breath work and meditation. What about meditation? Did Jesus meditate?

Yes, He did. Many times did Jesus go to be alone, away from the crowds, with his father, to pray and meditate.

Mark 1:35 (NIV) says, "Very early in the morning, while it was still dark, Jesus got up, left the house and went off to a solitary place, where he prayed."

Luke 5:15-16 (NIV) tells us, "Yet the news about him spread all the more, so that crowds of people came to hear him and to be healed of their sicknesses. But Jesus often withdrew to lonely places and prayed."

My view on meditation has changed: instead of emptying my mind, I fill it with Scripture. There are many ways to do this. Sometimes I just pick a Bible verse and read it repeatedly, then I pray about it and mediate on it.

There is a Bible habit called praying the Psalms where you go through the Psalms, one at a time, and pray over them. There are many different ways to meditate in a positive way that will not open doors to negative, harmful things.

Meditation has become widely recognized for its ability to ease stress and support emotional well-being—benefits that are especially valuable during perimenopause. Research has shown that meditation impacts both the mind and body by calming the neuroendocrine system and reducing immune-related stress responses.

A pivotal study by Pace et al. demonstrated that compassion meditation can actually downregulate the body's innate immune response to stress. In simple terms, this means meditation doesn't just help you feel calmer—it biologically reduces your body's overreaction to stress. This makes it a practical tool for managing chronic tension and mood fluctuations common in this season of life.

Walker's study of Jamaican school principals highlighted the value of combining mindfulness and prayer as a coping strategy for stress and anxiety. Participants reported that spiritual practices like meditation offered a sense of serenity and clarity during emotionally demanding times. This resonates with many women who are seeking tools to stay centered through hormonal shifts and life transitions.

In a clinical setting, Hatmalyakin et al. found that mindfulness meditation significantly lowered stress levels among nurses in high-pressure ICU environments. Given the rise in burnout among healthcare professionals, these results are a powerful reminder that mindfulness can restore emotional resilience even in the most demanding circumstances.

Likewise, a study by Duraimani found that using a mobile app to guide daily meditation led to reduced anxiety and better workplace satisfaction. Employees reported feeling more capable and emotionally balanced—further proving that structured mindfulness can be easily integrated into a busy lifestyle with real, lasting benefits.

Finally, Sadowski et al. showed that those who practiced meditation had lower salivary cortisol levels—a biological marker of stress—and reported a noticeable drop in perceived tension. This ties the emotional and physiological benefits of meditation together, offering concrete evidence of its power to support whole-body peace.

Together, these studies make a strong case: meditation isn't merely an optional practice—it's a scientifically supported, spiritually grounding tool to help women thrive through perimenopause.

What About the Vagus Nerve?

The vagus nerve is a powerful, often overlooked, tool for healing—especially for women in midlife. Think of it as the brake pedal of your nervous system. While your sympathetic nervous system revs you up to fight, freeze, or flee, your vagus nerve activates your parasympathetic system, which tells your body, *"You're safe now—it's time to rest, digest, and repair."*

The word vagus comes from Latin, meaning "wandering," and that's exactly what it does—it wanders through your body, connecting your brain to your gut, heart, lungs, and more. It's the main communication highway that governs everything from your mood to your metabolism.

Stimulating the vagus nerve can profoundly impact your:

- hormonal balance (especially during perimenopause)
- immune system regulation (key in autoimmunity and inflammation)
- gut-brain communication
- emotional resilience (through its influence on anxiety, mood, and sleep)

When your vagus nerve is functioning well—what we call having good vagal tone—your body can better handle stress, regulate hormones, and recover from daily demands. When it's underactive, you may experience things like poor digestion, heightened anxiety, brain fog, or a constant state of wired-but-tired exhaustion.

Benefits of Vagus Nerve Stimulation:

- Lowers inflammation by turning on your body's anti-inflammatory reflex
- Supports balanced cortisol and progesterone levels
- Improves digestion and motility (especially helpful in bloating and constipation)
- Enhances emotional regulation and reduces anxiety
- Promotes deeper sleep and improved recovery

Cultivate Simple Practices for the Vagus Nerve

In perimenopause, when your body is already under hormonal stress, activating your vagus nerve is essential. You can't supplement your way out of stress if your nervous system is stuck in survival mode. But with small, intentional practices, you can begin to reset your system and signal to your body: *You're safe now. Let's heal.*

You can gently stimulate your vagus nerve through several simple, daily practices:

- Breathwork is one way to shift your body into a parasympathetic state.
- Gargling or humming activates the throat muscles and vocal cords, directly stimulating vagal pathways.
- Similarly, singing—whether it's worship music or breath prayers—stimulates the vagus nerve through vibration in the vocal cords.
- Cold exposure, like splashing cold water on your face or ending a shower with cool water, activates the vagal reflex and can lower stress signaling.
- Regular prayer and meditation increase parasympathetic tone while calming the overactive HPA (stress) axis.
- Laughter and meaningful social connection also stimulate vagus activity by boosting oxytocin and emotional safety.

- For some individuals, vagal nerve stimulation devices (like TruVaga) offer targeted stimulation and are also used clinically in conditions like migraines, depression, and inflammatory disorders.

BREATHWORK BASICS

4-7-8 breathwork

This technique regulates the autonomic nervous system by activating the parasympathetic nervous system (PNS)—the "rest and digest" mode that counters fight-or-flight sympathetic nervous system responses.

HOW TO DO THE 4-7-8 BREATHING TECHNIQUE

Step 1: Sit comfortably with a straight back, or lie down in a relaxed position.

Step 2: Place the tip of your tongue against the roof of your mouth (just behind your upper teeth) and keep it there until exhale.

Step 3: Inhale deeply through your nose for 4 seconds.

Step 4: Hold your breath for 7 seconds.

Step 5: Exhale slowly and completely through your mouth for 8 seconds, making a "whoosh" sound.

Step 6: Repeat this cycle at least 3 times (or more if needed).

BOX BREATHING

Box breathing is another breathwork technique. You take a breath in, hold, breathe out, and hold. Repeat until calm.

Praying the Psalms

Use the Psalms as a source of comfort, strength, and connection. Psalms like Psalm 23 and Psalm 91 offer reassurance in difficult times, while Psalm 139 emphasizes God's intimate knowledge and love for each person.

> Be still, and know that I am God:
> I will be exalted among the heathen, I will be exalted in the earth.
>
> —Psalm 46:10 (KJV)

What about hitting valleys and hard times?
Why did God do this to me? you may ask.

Just as lifting weights tears down muscle so it can rebuild stronger, God uses trials to refine our faith and deepen our dependence on Him. These hard seasons are not wasted; they are part of His sovereign plan to shape you into a women who is steadfast, humble, and anchored in His grace—not merely your own strength.

> Think over what I say, for the Lord
> will give you understanding in everything.
>
> —2 Timothy 2:7 (ESV)

When I was practicing yoga regularly and teaching it, I kept asking other Christians, "Is this okay?" I don't think I was asking the correct questions. I also think that sometimes it's hard to call people out. This yoga discussion is very controversial, and I don't know why. It gets heated when you post about it online.

When I felt convicted, I posted my views about yoga on social media. Mostly I heard amazing testimony in response, including a former studio owner who felt convicted by the Holy Spirit to terminate her business. Others who said they never could get into yoga were most likely being protected from it. Others such as yoga studio owners were attacking me and calling me names on my Facebook account. I believe they felt condemned and were taking it out on me.

I once said that yoga was healing people. Now, the only healing I want is from the healer, Jesus. Anything else comes at the price of your soul.

I look back at that time in my life and I wasn't at peace. I was a Christian, but I wasn't living in the Word—more like living in the world.

My identity during most of my 30s was tied up as a doctor, a mother, a yoga instructor, and a small business owner, while it should have been focused on the fact that I am a daughter of the King.

If you went down this path, as I did, while trying to find natural solutions to your perimenopause problems, look at my testimony.

Chapter Key Takeaways:

- New Age practices aren't true healing. Seek to build a stronger relationship with God and watch true peace and healing unfold.
- You can improve stress resilience by adopting breath work and meditation.
- Begin integrating vagus nerve practices into your routine because it helps regulate everything from your mood to your hormones.

CHAPTER 9

Cultivate a Deep Relationship with God

> He who was seated on the throne said, "I am making everything new!" Then He said, "Write this down, for these words are trustworthy and true."
>
> —Revelation 21:5 (NIV)

Cultivating a spiritual relationship with Jesus does take time out of your day, but I'll make it easy for you to start. First, fill your mind with the good stuff. We spoke about this earlier on in the book—filling your mind with things that are good—why would you fill it with bad stuff? Those bad things are certainly from the enemy.

You know what's beautiful about the Holy Spirit? He speaks—gently, clearly, and always in love. When you learn to listen, He'll guide you, help you, and remain by your side in every season.

I remember one quiet evening, sitting in my bathtub, reading and soaking while listening to worship music. In that stillness, I felt a nudge—one that could only come from the Spirit—urging me to talk to my son about something important. It wasn't loud. It wasn't forced. Just a gentle whisper on my heart.

That's how He moves. Like when a friend randomly pops into your thoughts—don't brush it off. Call them. Pray for them. Follow the prompting.

Learning to discern the Holy Spirit's guidance is like exercising a muscle: over time, as you trust, obey and stay anchored in God's Word, your spiritual sensitivity grows stronger and clearer.

Reading the Bible

You have access to God's Word—don't let it sit unopened. Make time for it daily. You'll never regret the moments you spend in Scripture. Honestly, it's a far better habit than doomscrolling, and it actually brings peace instead of anxiety.

> Your Word I have treasured and stored in my heart,
> That I may not sin against You.
>
> —Psalms 119:11 (AMP)

I committed to reading the Bible in a year. I found that the book and podcast series called *The Bible Recap* is a great resource. I would listen to it all on my phone. I would have no excuses at all for not focusing on it. I love to listen to the recap and the Scripture while lifting weights or going for a walk. It would bring such joy to me. Along with two faith-based books a month plus discussions with friends, I experienced a deeper awareness of the Holy Spirit's work in my life.

We need to start lifting our spiritual muscles. What if you lift weights but are not using the right building blocks? If you don't provide your body with protein and amino acids after your workout, you won't build new muscle. If you want to be spiritually strong, you need the correct foundation, which is spending time with the Lord and reading your Bible.

Sarcopenia is when your muscles waste away. I see many with a sarcopenic spirit; they let different idols of the world—like their career, wealth, status, and material things—take over as an idol in their life. This way, they waste away instead of building up and becoming strong.

> But very truly I tell you, it is for your good that I am going away.
> Unless I go away, the Advocate will not come to you;
> but if I go, I will send him to you.
>
> —John 16:7 (NIV)

Jesus is talking about the Holy Spirit. We are never alone, since the Holy Spirit dwells here on earth with us. The Holy Spirit in the AMP Bible version is called the Helper, Comforter, Advocate, Intercessor, Counselor, Strengthener, and Standby.

Wait, what? I was looking at crystals, practicing reiki, and burning sage when I had the Holy Spirit with me? I wasn't tapping in and spending time with Him anymore. The enemy had me distracted, and I fell for it. A lot of us fall for it, because it's hard and we live in a broken world. The more I think about it, it seems to me that we are not prepared, and we are not ready for battle. We need to start lifting those spiritual muscles.

10 Minutes With Him: Strong And Anchored In Jesus

3 Minutes of Praise/Worship Song: Start each day by listening to a worship song to set a positive tone and focus on gratitude. Praise music can remind you of God's goodness and provide an uplifting start to the day.

3 Minutes in Scripture: Read a short passage from the Bible to gain wisdom, encouragement, or insight. Choose a verse or chapter that resonates with current challenges or goals.

2 Minutes in Prayer: Spend two minutes in personal prayer, sharing your concerns, expressing gratitude, and seeking guidance. Keep it simple and honest, focusing on connecting with God.

1 Minute of Gratitude: Close with a minute reflecting on things you're grateful for, big or small. Gratitude shifts focus away from stressors and promotes a positive mindset to carry throughout the day. Praise God for all your blessings.

1 Minute in Silence, Listening to the Holy Spirit: Use this time to quiet your mind and be receptive to any insight or encouragement from the Holy Spirit.

You can use a journal for these ten minutes. Cuddle up with a blanket in the early morning and set your intentions toward Jesus for the day. This is powerful. We know that to truly know Him, we need to spend time with Him. Set your morning with the intention to give your day to Jesus, knowing that He is in control. You can repeat this 10-minute habit with Him a few times a day.

10 Minutes with Him:
Strong and Anchored in Jesus

3 Minutes of Praise/Worship Song:
Start each day by listening to a worship song to set a positive tone and focus on gratitude.

3 Minutes in Scripture:
Read a short passage from the Bible to gain wisdom, encouragement, or insight.

2 Minutes in Prayer:
Spend two minutes in personal prayer, sharing your concerns, expressing gratitude, and seeking guidance.

1 Minute of Gratitude:
Close with a minute reflecting on things you're grateful for, big or small. Praise God for all your blessings.

1 Minute in Silence:
Listening to the Holy Spirit.

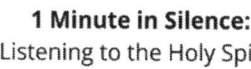

Connect with Truth: Planting a Seed of Connection with God

What if you feel rejected? Have patience, and remember your worth and security are anchored in Christ alone. Even when people fail you, God's covenant and love does not change. In seasons of loneliness, lean on His promises and trust that He is working all things for your good and His glory.

> The stone the builders rejected
> has become the cornerstone.
>
> —Matthew 21:42 (CSB)

What is your identity? For a long time, I believed my identity was wrapped up in my titles—first as a doctor, then as a mother. But the truth is that neither of those roles define who I am at my core. They are blessings, yes—beautiful assignments from God—but they are not my identity.

It took time (and some holy conviction) to realize I had been building my sense of self on worldly things. And while those things may bring temporary purpose, they can never bring lasting peace.

My true identity? I am a daughter of the King. That's it. That's everything.

When we root our identity in Jesus, joy can't be stolen, no matter what role we hold or what season we're in. Our work, our relationships, even our ministries—they're gifts. But they aren't who we are.

Surround yourself with people who will remind you of that. People who live biblically, who pray with you, who point you back to truth.

And here's one daily habit that helps: Spend ten minutes with Him. Just ten minutes—listening, reading, praying. That's all it takes to plant a seed of connection that God will water and grow.

> I planted the seed, Apollos watered the plants, but God made you grow. It's not the one who plants or the one who waters who is at the center of this process but God, who makes things grow.
>
> —1 Corinthians 3:6–7 (MSG)

Prayers: Encourage setting intentions at the beginning of each day, week, or month, focusing on gratitude, positivity, and faith. You can also ask God for help through personal prayers—praying about family goals, support for the community, and whatever else you need to pray for. Write them down and then reflect later in the month on how God provides. My family hangs on our door a prayer request as "Please" and answered prayers as "Thank you" (from the movie *Unsung Hero*). It's so beautiful to watch God work in our daily lives.

> Ask and it will be given to you; seek and you will find; knock and the door will be opened to you.
>
> —Matthew 7:7 (NIV)

Journaling: Documenting reflections, prayers, or moments of gratitude can deepen the connection with yourself and God.

> They speak of the glorious splendor of your majesty—
> and I will meditate on your wonderful works.
>
> —Psalm 145:5 (NIV)

Community: Engage with like-minded individuals or small groups to stay motivated, share experiences, and deepen spiritual growth together. God wants us not to be isolated, but to live in community. It's not always easy. Community can be messy, trying, and imperfect. But it is also refining, healing, and deeply biblical. When we isolate, we become easier targets for spiritual attack. But when we walk in unity, we reflect the body of Christ.

So lean in. Join the study. Go to the gathering. Text that friend. Don't do life alone.

> And though one can overpower him who is alone,
> two can resist him.
> A cord of three strands is not quickly broken.
>
> —Ecclesiates 4:12 (AMP)

So that Christ may dwell in your hearts through faith.
And I pray that you, being rooted and established in love.

—Ephesians 3:17 (NIV)

Things that can trap you: tarot cards, fortune telling, yoga, reiki, energy work

Think: if it's not rooted in Christ, stay away: it's only going to bring darkness into your life.

Spiritual Warfare

I went to a conference last December, by myself. Usually I meet a friend, share a room, or bring one of my children. This was a quick trip for networking and preparing for the release of this book.

While I prayed about coming, I finally booked the flight and the hotel. Well, I got sick. It's bizarre because I had been sleeping, taking all the supplements, all the peptides, and trying to manage stress. This isn't like me. I could muscle through it, but I lost my voice. Yep. My voice that I needed to network.

Worse yet, as I sat in the bathtub alone, I started hearing those thoughts. You know the ones.

You are not good enough. You are a failure. No one likes you. This book is going to do badly. You can't shift integrative/functional medicine away from the New Age. Why did you leave your family to come here?

These thoughts are not from God! They are from the enemy. This was a spiritual battle, and I was caught off guard.

> Keep a cool head. Stay alert. The Devil is poised
> to pounce and would like nothing better than to catch
> you napping. Keep your guard up. You're not the
> only ones plunged into these hard times.
> It's the same with Christians all over the world.
> So keep a firm grip on the faith.
> The suffering won't last forever.
> It won't be long before this generous God
> who has great plans for us in Christ—
> eternal and glorious plans they are—will have
> you put together and on your feet for good.
> He gets the last word; yes, he does.
>
> —1 Peter 5:8–11 (MSG)

If we let the enemy's thoughts fill our mind, we will start to believe these things. Has this happened to you? When you have a setback and suddenly you are on the couch, eating a bag of chips, ready to throw in the towel.

I believe the enemy preys on women in perimenopause. With our hormones fluctuating, many going through transition of jobs, children, and aging parents, we are an easy target to take down. Also, if you are sharing your faith, you are in the arena, and that makes the enemy mad. But guess what? Jesus has more power. I will help show you how to use that power!

My goodness, I picked up the book I brought with me, turned on praise music, sent a text to my prayer warriors, and told the enemy he will not win!

The battle is spiritual.

At the end of my time at the conference, I took the red-eye home Saturday night to get baptized on Sunday. Was the devil ever mad! I smiled and laughed at this as I wrote this section in the city of sin: Las Vegas.

As I wrote this, I paused to thank God for leading me to share this chapter on spiritual health in perimenopause. I've walked through it myself, and I can tell you with certainty—He has already won the battle. Your strength doesn't have to come from within. It comes from Jesus. All you need to do is receive it.

Chapter Key Takeaways:

- Strengthen your walk with Christ by reading scripture regularly.
- Spend ten minutes with Him: anchor your connection through prayer, scripture, and listening
- Battle spiritual warfare—tune out the enemy and trust in the power of Jesus

CHAPTER 10

Cycle Syncing

Your Hormone-Smart Guide to Navigating
the Menstrual Cycle in Perimenopause

I have used cycle syncing for years in my office, positioning women for success from their teens to perimenopause. It's a beautiful way to connect with your God-given menstrual cycle. Using the natural rhythm of our cycling hormones, we can adjust our diet, exercise, and even social habits to our cycle, setting us up for victory instead of frustration.

Did you know there are times in your cycle when you are going to be able to fast more successfully or are less likely to get injured at the gym?

There are also studies to indicate that women are move creative when they are most fertile. Leading up to ovulation might be a great time to brainstorm or make creative decisions.

For a refreshing recap on the menstrual cycle feel free to go back to the introduction.

Diet: Eating for Your Cycle

The menstrual cycle is a complex interplay of hormones that influences various physiological processes, including metabolism, appetite, and energy utilization.

Recent studies suggest that dietary patterns, particularly the adoption of a ketogenic diet during the follicular phase and increasing carbohydrate intake during the luteal phase, may align with the body's hormonal fluctuations. Research indicates that during the follicular phase, women may experience enhanced fat oxidation, making a ketogenic diet—high in fats and low in carbohydrates—potentially beneficial. The increased insulin sensitivity observed during this phase supports the utilization of fat as a primary energy source, aligning with the metabolic adaptations induced by a ketogenic diet.

Follicular Phase

- Protein: Pastured eggs, grass-fed beef, wild-caught salmon, sardines
- Healthy fats: Avocado, extra-virgin olive oil, coconut oil, ghee
- Nuts & seeds: Macadamia nuts, walnuts, chia, flaxseed
- Non-starchy vegetables: Leafy greens, broccoli, cauliflower, zucchini, asparagus
- Fermented foods: Sauerkraut, kimchi
- Bone broth: Rich in collagen and minerals

Following ovulation, the luteal phase is marked by elevated progesterone levels, which can lead to increased appetite and cravings for carbohydrates. Progesterone is known to influence energy metabolism, often resulting in a higher basal metabolic rate (BMR) and increased caloric needs. BMR is the number of calories your body needs to perform its most basic functions. During this phase, women may benefit from a higher carbohydrate intake to meet these energy demands and alleviate cravings.

Luteal Phase

- Protein: Free-range poultry, fatty fish, grass-fed beef, eggs
- Healthy fats: Avocado, olives, raw nuts, nut butters
- Moderate carbs: Pumpkin, carrots, beets
- Magnesium-rich foods: Dark chocolate (85%), pumpkin seeds, leafy greens
- Fiber-rich veggies: Brussels sprouts, cabbage, green bean
- Berries: raspberries, blackberries, strawberries

Leptin is a hormone made by fat cells that tells your brain when you're full and helps regulate metabolism. High leptin means less hunger, while low leptin means more hunger.

During the follicular phase, lower leptin levels may correlate with reduced appetite and caloric intake. The ketogenic diet, which often leads to weight loss and decreased body fat, may further lower leptin levels, promoting fat utilization for energy. This aligns with findings that suggest women may naturally consume fewer carbohydrates during this phase, as their bodies are primed for fat metabolism. This is why I recommend fasting during this phase or a low-carb, ketogenic diet.

In contrast, leptin levels tend to rise during the luteal phase, which can contribute to increased appetite and cravings for carbohydrates. The rise in leptin may be a response to the increased energy demands associated with higher progesterone levels. Consuming more carbohydrates during this phase can help manage these cravings and support energy needs, as carbohydrates can stimulate insulin release, which in turn can enhance leptin sensitivity.

This is why I recommended a gentle increase in carbs during the luteal phase, if a patient's body is asking for it. If patients want to continue lower carb, I have them increase healthy fats. What I don't want is women to be binging on processed carbs during this phase or restricting their body and stressing it out (producing more cortisol, which can decrease progesterone).

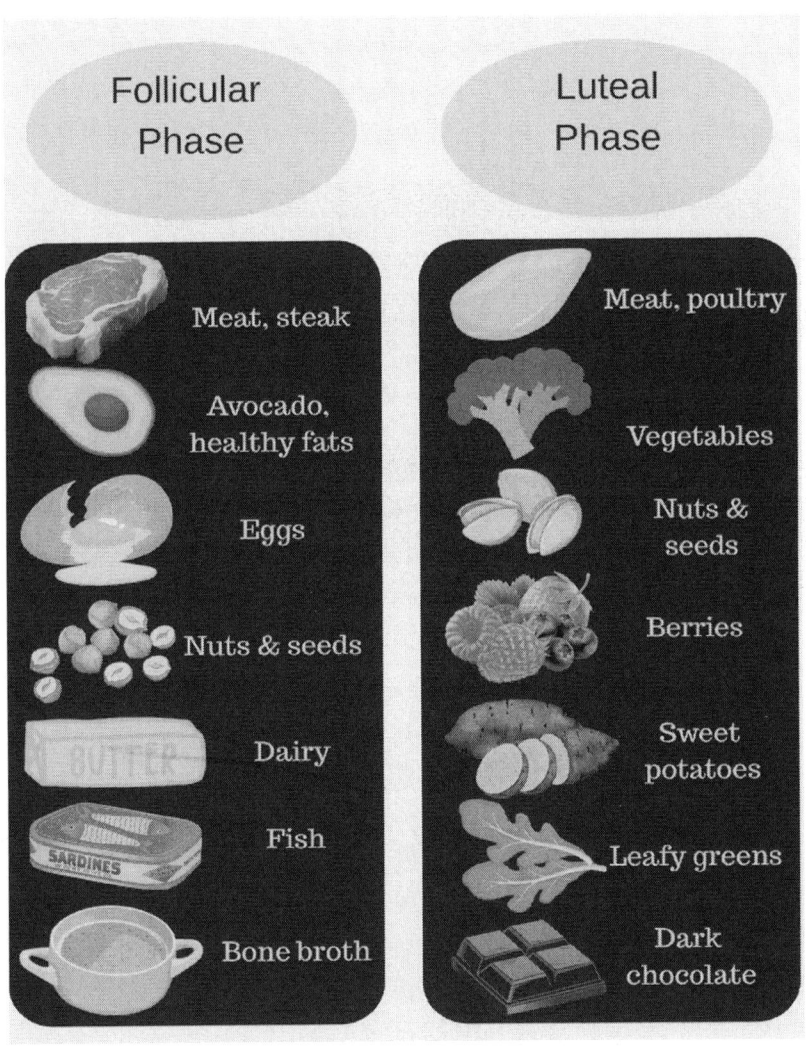

When women are more in tune with their cycle and how they are eating they, can be confident in food choices and not feel shame when eating carbs during the luteal phase. A ketogenic diet during the follicular phase may enhance fat utilization and stabilize blood sugar levels, while increased carbohydrate intake during the luteal phase can address cravings, support energy needs, and improve mood.

Recently, I was visiting my parents in Florida. While I am always on the hunt for protein and healthy fats, I was also just eating a lot more carbs. My dad noticed my appetite, so I discussed the luteal phase and cycle syncing with him. I was not worried about "overdoing it" on carbs, as I knew I would most likely be fasting and in ketogenesis (when your liver turns fat into ketones for energy instead of using carbs) during my follicular phase.

Are you feeling heard right now? Are you shaking your head in agreement and sick of restricting, then binging? Maybe you are doing that because you try to fast in the wrong part of your cycle, and you are fighting your hormones. I would not recommend this, because that, my friend, is a losing battle.

> ### How Estrogen and Progesterone Affect Blood Sugar
>
> Estrogen → Improves Insulin Sensitivity (Lowers Blood Sugar)
>
> - Estrogen helps insulin work more efficiently, allowing cells to further absorb glucose easily.
> - This results in lower blood sugar levels and better blood sugar control.
> - It also reduces fat storage and promotes the use of glucose for energy, keeping metabolism balanced.
>
> Progesterone → Can cause Insulin Resistance (Raises Blood Sugar)
>
> - Progesterone makes cells less responsive to insulin, leading to mild insulin resistance.
> - This means glucose stays in the bloodstream longer, causing higher blood sugar levels.
> - It also encourages fat storage and increases hunger, as the body prepares for a possible pregnancy—ensuring enough energy is available if fertilization occurs!
>
> I always recommend to patients when utilizing a CGM that they wear it their entire cycle because our sensitivity to insulin changes.

The Menstrual Cycle and Exercise: Sync Your Workouts

The menstrual cycle can impact physical performance and recovery. Cycle syncing can help women tailor their workout routines to align with their hormonal fluctuations.

During the follicular phase, we experience improved energy levels and performance, making it an ideal time for strength training and endurance workouts. Estrogen has been shown to positively influence muscle repair and recovery, making this an optimal time for high-intensity interval training workouts (HIIT and sprint intervals) and strength training. Research indicates that women may be more resilient to injuries during this phase.

During the luteal phase, women may experience a decrease in exercise performance and an increased risk of injury. Studies have shown that women are more susceptible to injuries during the luteal phase, potentially due to hormonal fluctuations affecting muscle and joint stability. It is advisable to avoid HIIT (high intensity interval training) workouts during this time.

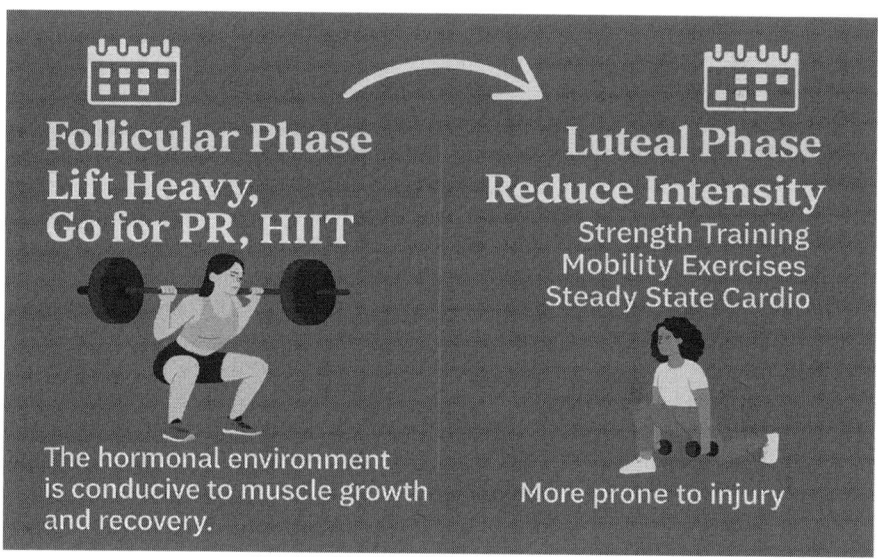

Adding in seed cycling can also be beneficial. When specific seeds are incorporated into the diet at different phases of the menstrual cycle, seed cycling provides essential nutrients that help modulate estrogen and progesterone levels. During the follicular phase (days 1–14), flax and pumpkin seeds, which are rich in lignans, omega-3s, and zinc, support estrogen production and prepare the body for progesterone secretion. In the luteal phase (days 15–28), sesame and sunflower seeds offer lignans, omega-6s (which convert to gamma-linolenic acid), and selenium, aiding in hormone regulation and detoxification of excess hormones.

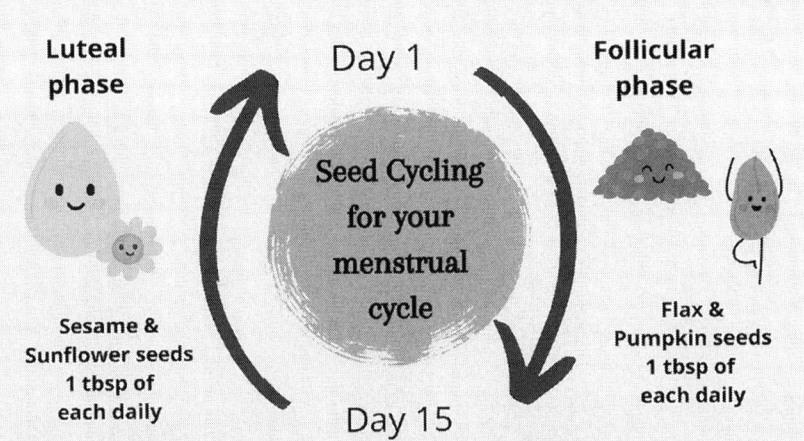

Flax seeds contain lignans, plant compounds that help modulate estrogen levels. If estrogen is too high, lignans can bind excess estrogen and help clear it. If estrogen is low, they have mild phytoestrogenic effects that gently support production.

Pumpkin seeds are rich in zinc, which supports healthy follicle development in the ovary and can help regulate estrogen and progesterone later.

Zinc also promotes proper pituitary signaling (FSH and LH).

Sesame seeds have higher lignan content and important minerals (like zinc and selenium) that help clear excess estrogen, creating better balance for progesterone to rise.

Sunflower seeds are rich in vitamin E, a nutrient shown to support corpus luteum function (the structure that produces progesterone after ovulation).

Vitamin E can also help reduce PMS symptoms and support luteal phase hormone levels.

Track Your Success!

Before you start your 28-day journey, take some measurements. Weigh yourself and take a waist-to-hip ratio (WHR).

To calculate your waist-to-hip ratio, you'll need a flexible measuring tape. Start by measuring your waist at the narrowest part, just above the belly button and below the rib cage. Stand relaxed, exhale gently (without sucking in your stomach), and wrap the tape snugly around your waist, ensuring it remains parallel to the floor. Next, measure your hips at the widest point, usually around the buttocks or hip bones, while keeping your feet together. Divide your waist measurement by your hip measurement to get your WHR.

> According to the World Health Organization (WHO), a WHR of 0.80 or below for women and 0.95 or below for men indicates a low risk for metabolic diseases. A WHR above 0.86 in women or 1.0 in men suggests a higher risk of cardiovascular disease, diabetes, and other health concerns. Since abdominal fat is more metabolically active, a higher WHR is associated with a greater risk of insulin resistance and chronic inflammation.

CYCLE SYNCING REVIEW:

- Follicular Phase: Focus on Strength Training. Utilize this phase to engage in high-intensity workouts, strength training, and endurance exercises. The hormonal environment is conducive to muscle growth and recovery.
- Luteal Phase: Reduce Intensity. Focus on moderate-intensity exercises, such as steady-state cardio, strength training, mobility exercises, or Pilates, which can help manage fatigue and mood swings.
- The focus during all phases should be weightlifting, with heavier weights and fewer reps in the follicular phase, and lighter weights but more reps in the luteal phase.

It is also important to get your husband and family on board with this! They will start to be more aware of why you might be acting a certain way on a specific day. Remember: male hormones have a 24-hour cycle, while women's hormones have a 28-day cycle. Check out the chart below as it will be very useful to help you stay on track.

PHASE	DURATION (DAYS)	HORMONE LEVELS	ACTIVITIES & PRE-CAUTIONS	NUTRITION
Menstrual Phase	1-4	Low estrogen & progesterone	Gentle exercise (e.g., walking, stretching). Time for reflection & evaluation. CLEANSE	Can be lower carb, plenty of electrolytes and hydration. Iron-rich foods/supplements.
Follicular Phase	5-14	Rising estrogen, surge in LH (luteinizing hormone) and FSH (follicle stimulating hormone) before ovulation	Optimal for brainstorming, starting projects, high-energy tasks. Ideal for strength training (make PRs) or cardio (HIIT & sprints) and social interactions. CREATE	Best time for Keto/Fasting: this is where you would do your longer fasts. Fiber-rich veggies and nuts. Macros: <50 C, 120-150 P, 120-180 F
Ovulation	Around Day 14	Peak in estrogen, surge in LH	Ideal for social interactions and intercourse (with pregnancy risk). Glowing, take pictures, make appearances, give presentations. COLLABORATE	Can be lower carb, no long fasts
Luteal Phase	15-28	Rising then falling progesterone, declining estrogen	Suited for focused, lower-energy tasks & project completion. Less inclination for social interactions. Increased risk of injury as menstruation nears. CULTIVATE	Add in complex carbs, certain veggies, prebiotics. Avoid simple/processed carbs. Macros: 1 100-150 C, 120 P, 80 F

And we know that for those who love God all things work together for good, for those who are called according to his purpose.

—Romans 8:28 (ESV)

So, ladies, I encourage you to start slow and follow this hormone-smart guide to help you feel your best! Cycle syncing can do wonders not only for your body, but for your mind and spirit too.

When you sync your diet and workouts with your cycle, notice how balanced, peaceful, and joyful you feel. God has created you with purpose and the capacity to thrive.

Take that first step. Cycle syncing isn't about perfection—it's about honoring how God made you and trusting Him to guide you into greater well-being and health.

Chapter Key Takeaways:

- A low-carb diet that is high in fats is best during the follicular phase
- Eat complex carbs during the luteal phase
- Utilize cycle syncing to align your exercise routines with your hormonal fluctuations

Part 4:
28-Day Plan and Devotional

Before you dive in, I want to share what you'll find in the next pages. The 28-day plan is here to guide you step by step toward better health, with daily actions you can put into practice—simple nutrition tweaks, lifestyle habits, and mindset shifts to help you feel more like yourself again. Alongside the plan, you'll also find a 28-day devotional. I wrote it openly and honestly, as a woman walking through perimenopause myself. My hope is that these reflections and Scriptures will encourage your heart, remind you you're not alone, and help you draw strength from the Lord as you begin this journey.

Your 28-Day Plan to Energize Your Body, Shed Weight, and Find Peace with God

Week 1

Start on day 1 of your cycle. Download your free printable guide online here: www.healthybydrjen.com/theperimenopausereset

Environment:

Clean out your kitchen! Replace plastic containers with glass, silicone, or stainless steel.

Toss non-stick cookware and use stainless steel or cast iron.

Body:

Eliminate gluten from your diet, 100%. Start today!

Start lifting weights: Three to four times a week for 30 minutes. On off-days, incorporate sprints during the follicular phase.

Spirit:

Every day, practice 10 Minutes with Him: Strong and Anchored in Jesus.

I recommend waking up 10 minutes earlier and starting your morning with this practice. Don't know which scripture to start with? Praying and meditating over the Psalms are a great place to start.

Week 2

ENVIRONMENT:

Clean out your laundry room. Swap your scented laundry soap with natural soap. Ditch the dryer sheets and use wool dryer balls with essential oils.

Avoid blue light at night. Put the phone down, get some red light or candlelight, and go to bed at a consistent time. Bonus: Track your sleep and aim for two hours of deep sleep.

BODY:

Try to incorporate fasting this week. Start with a 12-hour fast. If you already do this, extend it to 16 hours or even 24 hours. Try it out once if doing a 24-hour extended fast. Challenge: Try a 12-hour overnight fast every day this week!

SPIRIT:

Take inventory of the TV shows you watch, who you follow on social media, and the music you listen to. Cleanse all the negative input you have been exposing yourself to.

Week 3

ENVIRONMENT:

Examine your tap water at home. Make sure you have clean drinking water and proper filtration. Consider buying a whole-home filter or a tabletop filter system.

BODY:

Pay close attention to protein goals. Aim for 30 g with each meal and at least 120 g per day.

Continue lifting weights. On off-days, incorporate mobility stretching and walking during the luteal phase.

SPIRIT:

Chose a faith-based book to start reading with a group of friends. Set a date to discuss and share thoughts.

Week 4

ENVIRONMENT:

Look into your bathroom. Use shampoos without parabens and phthalates. Check your makeup for fragrances and toss out any cosmetics or perfumes that are questionable. Check personal care products to make sure they are unbleached, organic cotton.

BODY:

Wear a continuous glucose monitor. Start this week and wear it through a full cycle. Ensure you record everything you eat in the CGM app.

SPIRIT:

Make a prayer wall with your family where you put prayer requests up and pray together as a family. Continue 10 Minutes with Him.

Your Daily Cycle Day Devotional

Day 1

> So do not fear, for I am with you; do not be dismayed, for I am your God, I will strengthen you and help you; I will uphold you with my righteous right hand.
>
> —Isaiah 41:10 (NIV)

When we start a new month, we feel relief. We have been waiting (sometimes with symptoms) for the start of our cycle. For some who are trying to conceive, it's a sign of failure. I know it was for me.

When Chip and I got married, I was 29 years old, had just finished residency, and I was ready to be a mom. The plan was for me to be pregnant by age 30. Well, three cycles of trying went by and nothing. Meanwhile, I was taking a board review course in Vegas with a friend, and she was pregnant. I was so excited for her but also felt like a failure.

Little did I know, God was working with His timing and not mine. I was on birth control pills until I finally got off of them after my wedding—my body needed that time to detox.

Why the birth control? In high school, I was put on them to regulate my cycle (which really was a thyroid problem), and then the type A personality I was (I say *was* because I am a recovering type A personality now) liked the fact I could control exactly when I got my periods. The funny thing is that I always wanted to be in control of the timing of things in my life. In this case, I would have heard the whisper of *wait* if I had been listening.

The start of a new cycle means our hormones are all at the lowest point and the endometrium of our uterus is shedding, as no pregnancy occurred. This is a great time to take it easy as we start to get our energy back. These next few days it is best for you to take it slow.

Another tip is to look into your feminine products. Many can have toxic chemicals, like bleach, present. They even make tampons with fragrance in them! Fragrance is a word for hidden chemicals. What you want to look for is products with organic cotton. This would be pads and tampons. Another option is menstrual cups, or you can use cloth pads.

The fewer toxins in your body, the better for your hormone health. Chemicals in these products called xenoestrogens look like estrogens to our receptors. This means that they can really cause our hormones to spiral out of control with symptoms such as PMS, heavy periods, infertility, or short cycles.

While you are at it, throw away any plastic in your home that comes in contact with food. I know that it seems like a lot, but tiny switches will have big outcomes for your health.

A Prayer

Lord, thank you for this fresh start and new beginning. Let me trust You each month as You work all things for good. Amen.

Day 2

> Submit yourselves therefore to God.
> Resist the devil, and he will flee from you.
>
> —James 4:7 (ESV)

Tests are good. When we are tested, we need to hold onto our faith and praise, even in the valleys. Usually, tests are part of God's refinement processes.

I have personally felt this in my business. The hard seasons sometimes looked like falling to my knees, crying, and praying when things get difficult.

One fat that I love to use in my cooking is olive oil. It's very good for you! Did you know how olive oil is made? The olives are pressed and refined into oil. That pressing and stress actually result in something amazing.

Trust in the process. Sometimes you will feel crushed. That is where you undergo refinement. God is shaping and preparing you to become the best version of you. .

Always expect good things from God. You will have ups and downs in life. Don't let the tough moments make it seem like God is not righteous. He is good. He is perfect. He wants to give to us generously.

A PRAYER

Our heavenly father, I know You have had a plan from me since when You knitted me in my mother's womb. Help me see the valleys as times for pruning and growth so I can blossom and carry out Your plan for me. You are such a good God. Amen.

Day 3

> I can do all things through
> Him who gives me strength.
>
> —Philippians 4:13 (NIV)

"I can't do it anymore," I muttered under my breath while I picked up the fifth piece of gum on the ground from my four-year-old and stepped on a Lego. Ouch! (You all know it hurts!)

The enemy has a way to get into our mind when we are tired and weak. The devil waits around until we are running on low sleep and feeling rushed to make dinner, cleaning up the house, or shuffling kids to different activities. Can't you feel it? I want to remind you: You have the strength through Jesus.

When I notice the enemy trying to pick apart my marriage or my family, now I chuckle, say a prayer, or recite a scripture and take away those evil tactics. Haven't you ever noticed Sunday morning there is always bickering before church? Sometimes, it's hard to make it out the door on time, if at all. This comes from the enemy. Recognize this and fight back. You are strong and steady. Have faith in Jesus!

A PRAYER

Lord, You give me strength when I need it. I know You are always there to protect me, steadfast and unwavering. Help me to recognize when the enemy is going to attack, and help me use Scripture as a sword against the enemy. I know You are my strength and my shield. Amen.

Day 4

> Put on the full armor of God
> so that you can stand against the schemes of the devil.
>
> —Ephesians 6:11 (CSB)

One thing I will always be so grateful for is the time when I got bullied in 2022. That may sound odd. Before that, I didn't really know that spiritual warfare was real. During this time, I felt it. I experienced it. Without going through the hard time and leaning on my faith in Jesus, I would not have survived.

I came out of that season not just a stronger mother, friend, and woman—but a stronger follower of Christ. I'm more on fire for Jesus than ever before. I still have the screenshots of women cursing me and hoping I would fail. But instead of breaking me, it refined me. What the enemy meant for harm, God used to strengthen me into the very person they didn't want me to become.

One thing I've learned: The enemy can target those who walk in obedience. The bolder I became in my faith, the more intense the spiritual attacks became. But now I see them for what they are—confirmation that I'm walking the right path.

A PRAYER

Lord, thank you for Your armor against the enemy. The war has already been won, we just need to declare it. Give us strength from those that might cause us harm and help us stand firm against the devil's schemes. Amen.

Day 5

> So that it will not be obvious to others that you are fasting,
> but only to your Father, who is unseen,
> and your Father, who sees what is done in secret, will reward you.
>
> —Matthew 6:18 (NIV)

Have you ever fasted? Have you ever wanted to fast?

When I used to think of fasting, I didn't think it was something I could do! I also didn't realize that fasting can be abstaining from things other than food. I started a Sunday social media fast for 24 hours and I really have enjoyed it.

Fasting from food not only has spiritual benefits, but it also carries lots of health benefits with it. Short fasting, like overnight and 12 hours, gives lots of benefits for gut health. Our gut health is part of our immune system and needs to stay strong.

Making fasting a part of your monthly routine will help balance blood sugar, increase cellular autophagy (taking out the trash of our old and damaged cells), improve appetite control, and create mental clarity.

Picking when you fast is very important. Remember, the best time to do an extended food fast is in the follicular phase.

A prayer

Jesus, fasting and prayer shows our love to You and glorifies Your name. At time of fasting, let us spend that extra time with You in prayer. That time in prayer and scripture to get to know You better and take our eyes off worldly things. Amen.

Day 6

> Ask and it will be given to you; seek and you will find; knock and the door will be opened to you.
>
> —Matthew 7:7 (NIV)

In integrative medicine, I have my patients put the work in. When they have a breakthrough, they are so happy. I usually have tears in my eyes while praising their hard work.

See, they didn't just ask me for help with their health—they were seeking me out. When they arrived in my office they were clearly knocking on my door, ready and willing to commit to their health. My patients were aware of the time and financial obligations involved in caring for their hormone health.

I see this with our relationship with God. We need to knock on the door. This can mean developing your relationship with the Holy Spirit, fasting, observing the Sabbath, prioritizing church and time with God, or a mission trip showing your commitment to God. We think that just showing up for church every Sunday is enough. Start knocking!

A prayer

Jesus, please help me be committed to You. I want to knock so the door is open. My heart wants You to be first, and I long to be filled with the Holy Spirit. May I commit to You like I commit to so many other things and people. I know You are something worth knocking on all the doors for! Amen.

Day 7

> Daniel answered, "May the King live forever! My God sent his angel, and he shut the mouths of the lions. They have not hurt me, because I was found innocent in His sight. Nor have I ever done any wrong before you, Your Majesty."
>
> —Daniel 6:21–22 (NIV)

Being bold when it feels scary is hard. During the pandemic, I had to be bold. I had lives to save. I wasn't going to cower in the fear of what people would think. I knew that God would protect me as I came to rescue people. You know what He did? Not only did He protect me, but I also met some amazing people and saved many lives that otherwise would have perished in the hospitals.

Daniel in the lions' den trusted in God that he would be safe. God kept the lions' mouths shut so they did not harm him. Not one wound was found on him. That is the kind of trust I long to have for God.

Was I in the lions' den during the pandemic? Yes! I felt the pressure at times and still got backlash from my colleagues in conventional medicine, but ultimately I trusted in God that He would protect me. In Daniel's story, the king brought those who falsely accused Daniel to be thrown into the lion's den.

A prayer

Jesus, please show my heart Your everlasting power and help me trust that You are with me in the lions' den when I am doing Your work. Thank you for Your protection as I serve You. Amen.

Day 8

> So neither the one that plants nor the
> one who waters is anything,
> but only God, who makes things grow.
>
> —1 Corinthians 3:7 (NIV)

Early in my career as a business owner, all I thought about was how I could grow. How could I hire more instructors, get more clients, and bring in more money? Then COVID hit, and it all crumbled. As the founder of a small business, I didn't really get much help either.

Seeing patients is what kept my brick-and-mortar open during that time. We underwent a rebranding afterward. I noticed that my perception had also undergone a transformation. I was doing it all wrong. I was consulting everyone about my business, but not God.

How did this happen? I remember the day when I said *Lord, use me however you want: I am Yours*. After that, I had peace. I knew that now my business was in God's hands.

This surrender to God can also apply if you work for someone else or are a stay-at-home mom. We get so caught up in what we can build or do that we forget who is really in charge and who is guiding us. Once you give it back to God by placing your problems on the altar and putting Him in first place, the peace you will feel is astonishing.

A Prayer

Lord, use me as Your servant to spread Your love to others. My plans are not mine but Yours, and I am grateful I have You to consult with on any role or job I have. Let the Holy Spirit guide me daily through my life with work and family. Amen.

Day 9

> For I know the plans I have for you," declares the Lord,
> "plans to prosper you and not to harm you, plans to
> give you hope and a future.
>
> —Jeremiah 29:11 (NIV)

On my 42nd birthday, my children's school was cancelled because of a light snowfall (only two inches of snow). I had to laugh—growing up in Erie, Pennsylvania, we'd barely blink at that. On a snowy day there, it was common to have at least a foot of snow overnight. In Northwest Pennsylvania, even mentioning a snow day for anything less was a joke.

Normally, I'd be annoyed by such a mild-weather cancellation. But that day, I saw it as a gift. I had wanted to take the kids out to eat somewhere of their choosing, and now we wouldn't be rushed. I had been worried I wouldn't have enough time with them since my husband had made dinner plans with friends later that evening.

Of course, they picked Chick-fil-A—no surprise there! I brought along my Greek yogurt with added protein because I try to avoid seed oils. (I really wish they'd fry those waffle fries in tallow!)

Later that day, we heard about a volunteer opportunity at my son's school, and I was all in. The kids didn't hesitate either—they always jump in when I ask them to help, and they end up having the best time. All four of them got to work filling bags with beans and rice for children around the world.

Sure, I could have spent my birthday getting a massage, taking a girls' trip, or treating myself to a pedicure. But instead, I leaned into what God had for me that day—and it was so much better.

God has a plan for each day. Things that seem like a pain (snow day) are for a purpose. Lean into God's plan each day even in the moments when it feels hard.

A PRAYER

Lord, please mold my heart to trust You and be ready for an adventure You have planned for me, knowing that it is in Your perfect plan. Let me trust in Your sovereignty over every aspect of my life, the delays and cancellations, the victories and joy. You are so perfect and mighty. Amen.

Day 10

> Iron sharpens iron, and one man sharpens another.
>
> —Proverbs 27:17 (ESV)

Influence. Remember in Chapter 7 we discussed how you become like the five closest people you spend time with? What does this mean, exactly? The Bible holds a clue. Iron sharpens iron, and as 1 Corinthians 15:33 NIV says, "Do not be misled; bad company corrupts good character."

I have seen this at work. In a job my husband had, one employee talked behind everyone's back. This person tore others down, spread lies, and tried to make themselves look better by undermining coworkers and supervisors. My husband had to get out. It wasn't affecting his character, but it was causing him great stress. He tried to be positive, and we prayed for this person, but eventually he needed to cut it off.

Toxic workplaces, toxic friends, even toxic family members, can happen to anyone. Pray for discernment. Ask the Lord to put the right people in your life and pray for a change of those with hardest hearts.

A PRAYER

Jesus, we saw who was in Your circle of influence. We know Your character. I pray that You would surround me with people who love You, those who will sharpen my iron and point me to You. I ask if those in my circle are steering me away from the cross, that You soften their hearts and show them Your love. May You give me the clarity to see how those around me can influence me in a negative light, so I can be aware to use prayer and Scripture to turn on the lights in the darkness. I am so blessed to have You, Jesus, in my inner circle. Amen.

Day 11

> Finally, brothers, whatever is true, whatever is honorable, whatever is just, whatever is pure, whatever is lovely, whatever is commendable, if there is any excellence, if there is anything worthy of praise, think about these things.
>
> —Philippians 4:8 (ESV)

Have you ever started singing a song you heard many times on the radio and then realized that the lyrics were actually pretty revolting? And to make it worse, are your kids singing the lyrics also? Yes! This is when we switched the music we play in our home (and cars too) to Christian music on replay.

Christian music is good and uplifting. Have you tried listening? The best is when we are in our home or car and my children sing along. I know that God's Word is being hidden in their hearts. You never know when those words will be needed as your children leave the house.

A Prayer

God, give me wisdom when I choose what I listen to and input into my mind daily. Let me glorify Your name when I am singing music in the car, making dinner, or working out. Thank you for the blessings of Christian music and Your word. Amen.

Day 12

> For my yoke is easy, and my burden is light.
>
> —Matthew 11:30 (NIV)

Do you have burdens? Do you have stress? Or do you have peace and joy? What makes the difference? Giving your burdens to Jesus. He tells us to do so in the Bible. This doesn't mean we won't have a little stress—it's the pressure that makes the diamond—but to be burdened without hope is from the enemy.

I used to think I could fix everything and everyone. I am a doctor as well as a recovering type A personality, so this quirk can be accepted. I want to fix everyone's problems, no matter how big or small. By feeling this way, I also used to take on their burdens and internalize them.

How silly was I to think that I could do more about someone's problems than God. Ha! I laugh about it now. Oh, but when I write those prayers down, then I pray continuously, I see God working. Not my timing, but His glorious timing.

What do you do with your burdens? Give them to Jesus and feel that load lighten.

A prayer

Jesus, thank you for taking the burden from us and working to make all things good. It's such a blessing to know that You will take on the heavy. I know we are not guaranteed an easy life here on earth, but I can be less burdened if I ask You to live in my heart. What a great God you are to take on the burden, the hard things—we don't deserve it, but You do it anyway. Allow me to remember that You are the great physician, and only You can fix things that are broken. In Jesus' name. Amen.

Day 13

> But you must return to your God.
> Maintain love and justice and always put your hope in God.
>
> —Hosea 12:6 (CSB)

I was still a practicing Christian when I taught yoga and was a yoga studio owner. Post deliverance and repentance, I was convicted to stop all yoga, forever. I returned to God and gained the knowledge to save others from New Age practices that point us away from Jesus.

These practices can be incredibly deceptive. Many cling to them, placing all their hope in New Age customs that promise healing but often lead to deeper confusion and bondage. Out of both love and conviction, I speak out about how spiritually harmful they are. But I've also learned that discernment from God is essential—both in the timing and the way this truth is shared. It's not always easy, but I pray my testimony shines a light and brings clarity to those who need it.

A PRAYER

Lord, we can always return to You no matter what the sin or distraction. Jesus, You died for our sins. Help us to always point our eyes toward You and not get confused by the world. We love You and want to be in Your presence. Amen.

Day 14

> You intended to harm me, but God intended it for good
> to accomplish what is now being done, the saving of many lives.
>
> —Genesis 50:20 (NIV)

I was bullied. In 2022, a group of local moms were bullying me. They attacked my religious and medical views. It got so bad that I had to get the police involved. I would cry out, *Why, God? Why me?* It turned out that I was looking at it wrong. I didn't trust His plan.

I felt the whole experience pulling me closer to God, making me a stronger, better person. I came to the realization of how important it is to pray for those that hurt me, even if it was the last thing I wanted to do. (One of the bullies said they wanted me gone). It renewed my faith and made me push on. Praise in the valleys, and trust in God's plan!

A PRAYER

Lord, it can be tough to pray for those who hurt us. Sometimes, the last thing we want to do is to forgive those who harm us. Forgiveness brings us closer to You. Thank you for forgiving our sins. Let us forgive others. May the veils be lifted from their eyes and their hearts softened. Amen.

Day 15

> The righteous thrive like a palm tree and grow like a cedar tree in Lebanon. Planted in the house of the Lord.
>
> —Psalm 92:12 (NIV)

The perfect school, the best travel team, and the finest home is what we try to root ourselves in. We try to thrive and grow in the wrong places with mistaken intent. It's difficult to even realize we are doing this if we are hanging around the wrong people.

I was off course and not around believers, so I was planted in the garden box of the world, definitely not thriving. Following God's plan for us is how we can truly blossom and grow. It's difficult to realize what is important in life. It's time to slow down, begin to lead by example, and show your family what it means to be planted properly by the Lord and His word.

A Prayer

Jesus, You are the one who helps us grow when we feel like we are rooted in the wrong things, which will grow only shallow roots. Help us become righteous and grow deeply rooted in You so we may thrive like palm trees and grow like cedar trees. We are so thankful for the growth You bless us with when we follow You. In your name, Amen.

Day 16

> If you remain in me and my words remain in you,
> ask whatever you wish, and it will be done for you.
>
> —John 15:7 (NIV)

Do you ever feel like you take on too much? Yes, I will volunteer at the school, yes I will coach my son's basketball team, yes I will join that committee at work, yes I will plan the high school reunion. Now where does the time you spend with God daily come in?

I refer you to Part 3, where I discuss the 10 minutes with Him daily. Are you making this a priority? Start right when you wake up in the morning. This time spent with God will help you begin the day right.

It also helps to say "no" to things, so you can say "yes" to Jesus. He doesn't want you to do all the things. He wants you to spend time with Him and He wants your heart.

You don't have to give an automatic "yes" every time people ask you to do things. You can say, "I will get back to you," or "I am going to pray about it first."

Ask the Holy Spirit to guide you. It might not be a good season to do it all.

I remember one year I was running my business, volunteering on multiple boards, and coaching both a flag football team and a basketball team. Let me tell you, I didn't feel at peace. I felt rushed. This is not what God wants for us. Rather, He desires the opposite for us. He wants us to have time to rest.

A PRAYER

God, please allow me to say "no" to things that do not serve Your purpose. I know You want us to work hard on earth, but we should not be filling up our calendars with yeses just to be busy. Let me focus on the things You lead me to, and I pray for the discernment to know what I should say "yes" to and the things I should say "no" to. Jesus, I want to say "yes" to You all the time and put You first. This will set an example for my family and is the most biblical "yes" there is. Please give me peace and strength from the Holy Spirit as I say "no" to all the things and "yes" to You. In Jesus' name, Amen.

Day 17

> Aren't two sparrows sold for only a penny?
> But your Father knows when any one of them falls to the ground.
> So don't be afraid! You are worth much more than many sparrows.
>
> —Matthew 10:29–31 (CEV)

He's got you. Our God who looks after the sparrows and knows the number of hairs on your head. What a great God! (And that's something to remember, especially when we get that postpartum shed!) You are the daughter of a King. Jesus has got your back.

I know it seems like the days are long, but the years are short. Especially as mothers, we feel as though we give and don't receive. Think of this as a blessing: You get to serve every day and do it with joy, whether you are staying at home with your children or working outside of the household.

If you feel restless in your season, pray about it, and He will reveal His plan. The timing might not be your favorite, but He is going to guide you in the right direction.

A PRAYER

Lord, please give me comfort today knowing that You have my back. You always have the right timing. I know that even in the seasons or days of frustration that I should have a joyful heart. You know the hairs on my head, You look after the sparrows, You guide me daily if I open my heart to Your love. Thank you, Jesus, for the daily reminder of how special I am to You. Amen.

Day 18

> No temptation has overtaken you except what is common to mankind. And God is faithful; He will not let you be tempted beyond what you can bear. But when you are tempted, He will also provide a way out so that you can endure it.
>
> —1 Corinthians 10:13 (NIV)

"Here, take this crystal for protection. Put it in your pocket," the reiki master said. I went to three different sessions of reiki in total during my time in the New Age. It might be discomforting to discuss, but it happens to other Christians also. My reiki master professed she was Christian, but did I test this practice with the Bible?

My heart was tempted for healing that was beyond Jesus, and searching for power other than in the name of Jesus. That was dangerous, and it brought consequences at the expense of peace.

I praise God that He took me away and delivered me from the New Age practices. I felt as though I was in deep, but I wasn't. My heart still belonged to God. He provided not only a way out but a path forward—that I can be a light (in the darkness) to others who are tempted and misled.

A PRAYER

God, we are tempted daily to look outside of Your word for truth and to seek guidance other than Your voice. Thank you for bringing us out of temptation, delivering us from evil, and putting us back in Your open arms. Amen.

Day 19

> On the seventh day, God had completed His work that He had done, and He rested on the seventh day from all His work that He had done. God blessed the seventh day and declared it holy, for on it he rested from all His work of creation.
>
> —Genesis 2:2–3 (CSB)

Rest. As mothers, we tend to think of rest as only sleep. This needs to change because it's so much more than that. God rested, and He wants us to rest. Going nonstop all the time is hard on our body, specifically our adrenal glands. If we don't rest, we will end up doing damage to our body.

The other concern with the lack of rest that most of us experience is that it can affect our hormones, specifically progesterone. Let me, as a physician, give you permission to rest during your luteal phase. It is crucial.

When we rest, we allow our body to heal and work properly as God intended. If we don't rest, we disobey God, and we cause our bodies to weaken.

What does rest look like? Taking a walk outside in nature, soaking in an Epsom salt bath, or going to the coffee shop to read. Rest as He wants us to. Enjoy your family, your friends, and most importantly, your relationship with Jesus.

A PRAYER

Jesus, thank you for rest. Allow me to know when it's time to rest and when I need to take a sabbath as we are called to do. Allow me rest in Your arms, let me rest my mind if I work with my intellect all day, let me rest my body if I work with my hands all day. Even the animals do not work all day. Let me rest and refresh so that I may produce the good works that You have prepared for me. The dirty dishes and the messy playroom can wait. Lord, give me the strength to rest with my friends, family, and, most importantly, rest with You. In Jesus' name, Amen.

Day 20

> I call on the Lord in my distress, and He answers me.
>
> —Psalm 120:1 (NIV)

Why worry? I spent a lot of time worrying in my teens and 20s. I think back about what I could have been accomplishing instead of worrying.

Try to think of one time when being anxious and full of worry has made things better or helped a situation. Couldn't think of one, right? Do not be anxious but pray instead.

Many times, it's the last thing we do. Instead, we put on a reality TV show, scroll social media (doom scrolling) or shop online. Instead, we could open our Bible, call a friend to pray with us, read a devotional, or go on a nature walk while praying. Hold those anxious thoughts captive, and pray to your God.

A Prayer

Jesus, Your name holds the answer to peace. You abolish anxiety and fill our minds with comfort. Let us trust in You and You alone. Let us seek Your peace in our times of worry and anxiety. In Your precious name, Amen.

Day 21

> The words of the reckless pierce like swords,
> but the tongue of the wise brings healing.
>
> —Proverbs 12:18 (NIV)

I was crushed. I was on my knees bawling, crying out to God, *Why? What is your plan? I thought this was the plan!*

That day, I got a call from a friend who was supposed to join my brick-and-mortar practice. We had made all the plans, it was exciting, it was meant to happen. Until it wasn't.

I listened on the phone in shock. She asked if I had anything to say, but the Holy Spirit was whispering to me, *Be still.* Why? Because my heart was hurting, and if I spoke in that moment, my words would have cut, not healed. She didn't need my reaction—she already knew I was hurt. What she needed was my restraint. I didn't want to let my pain give birth to reckless words, when God was calling me to respond with wisdom and peace.

This friend had felt and heard God calling her to walk another path. How could I argue with that?

Praying over the disappointment was all I could do about it at that time—the pain I'd felt had melted away. I was so grateful for the Holy Spirit that day telling me to just be quiet at the right moment. I think we forget how much our words can hurt others and how much sin can come from the tongue. To this day, I'm thankful that I was able to listen.

A prayer:

God, please equip our ears to hear You, allow our tongues to pause and allow our hearts to trust You. You are the ultimate healer, and when we trust Your plan we will always have peace. Amen.

Day 22

The Lord is not slow in keeping his promise, as some understand slowness. Instead, He is patient with you, not wanting anyone to perish, but everyone to come to repentance.

—2 Peter 3:9 (NIV)

Stress can crush us sometimes. Nowadays everything and everyone is busy. We wake up, work out, get the kids ready for school, prepare ourselves for work, drop the kids off, go to the office, pick the kids up, make and eat dinner, take the kids to activities, arrive home, help with homework, and finally, it's bedtime.

Does this sound familiar? Are you rushed? Are you stressed? It's the sickness of busyness—we are too busy. I have four kids, so even when I don't overschedule, we are still bustling around just because of the number of children!

I have learned to slow down. Slowing down can still mean doing activities but doing them differently. Prioritizing the things that matter and letting go of the things that don't. Once you slow down, you can spend more time in the Word and in the presence of Jesus.

A prayer:

Lord, some think it's a badge of honor to be busy all the time, but it really just brings us further away from You. Help us to slow down and enjoy all the great things You bring us. Let us praise You with our most precious gift, our time. Amen.

Day 23

> And whatever you do, whether in work or deed,
> do it all in the name of Lord Jesus, giving thanks to God the Father through Him.
>
> —Colossians 3:17 (NIV)

My friend called me out.

She did. I was in her book club, and everyone was talking about Wednesday night church. We had recently started attending a church that had a Wednesday night service.

I said, "Oh yes, we can't do Wednesday because Cyrus has basketball and I really like this coach, so I didn't change the day and time." My friend said, "So you choose sports over God."

I was shocked, not at her saying those words, but that she spoke that bold, Spirit-led truth. But it was exactly what I needed to hear. From that moment on, I began planning our sports and activities around church.

Is it always perfect? No. Sometimes there are wrestling tournaments on Sundays, so we listen to church on the way there. What I'm asking is that you stay aware. Pay attention to where your time and energy are going. It all adds up—and it reflects what you truly value.

A Prayer

God, You should come first. Sometimes in this broken world we don't always see this. Let us see what is important and prioritize You as You prioritize us. Amen.

Day 24

> But if you are bitterly jealous and there is selfish ambition in your heart, don't cover up the truth with boasting and lying.
> For jealousy and selfishness are not God's kind of wisdom.
> Such things are earthly, unspiritual, and demonic.
>
> —James 3:14–16 (NLT)

What can the rushing women syndrome do to your health? It can affect your adrenal glands, your insulin levels, your thyroid health, and your hormones. It's a problem. What can help? Meditating on the Word.

I used to empty my mind when meditating. That is not the right approach. It's just asking for trouble. What is at the root of it all? Comparison to others, scrolling social media, and wondering how your life compares to others'.

Fill your mind with God's Word instead. Pick a verse or passage. Spend five to ten minutes reading it, and ask the Holy Spirit to reveal what you need to hear from it. This takes time and practice. Just like serving a volleyball or lifting weights, it takes time to flex this spiritual muscle.

Try it for the rest of the month: five to ten minutes a day of meditating on the Word. See how your mood changes. I also highly recommend adaptogens and L-theanine, which are great for adrenal support. Stay connected to God, even when you are busy.

A prayer

Jesus, let us slow down and worship You. Let us bask in Your light, which we need in the darkness of the everyday stresses we face day to day. You calm our soul and leave us rejuvenated. Amen.

Day 25

> For where you have envy and selfish ambition,
> there you will find disorder and every evil practice.
>
> —James 3:16 (NIV)

Comparison is the thief of joy. We hear that phrase a lot, and it is spot on. Comparison brings in sin: envy. We don't want or need that in our lives. It's different in today's world with social media when all we see is the highlight reel.

When I see some patients in my office, I am shocked at the trauma they have been through when I thought their lives were spotless. Some people go through so much pain but paint a perfect picture on their Christmas cards and social media.

This is the challenging thing about technology: it allows for constant comparison and a lack of empathy. We should not be envious or jealous of others. We should also not assume everything is perfect when someone could be struggling.

Have you ever felt this way? Everyone thinks you have it all together, but on the inside, you are wallowing in life's hardships. Find someone to talk to that you can confide in and open your heart to. There is one that is always there to search your heart—just talk with Him.

A Prayer

Lord, I know You are there, waiting to hear what is on my heart always. It's not always easy living in this broken world, but I know I can be real with You. Let me not compare my life or actions to others', but strive to be more like You, daily using the Bible as my guide. Thank you for always being there to listen to my cries and my celebrations. In Jesus' name. Amen.

Day 26

> Why are you down in the dumps, dear soul?
> Why are you crying the blues?
>
> —Psalm 42:5 (MSG)

Being vulnerable.

Usually around this day of my cycle is when I break down in tears once ... or twice. I know it's due to a major fluctuation of hormones, but it still happens occasionally.

Lean into it. Pray, journal, meditate on Scripture. Practice 10 minutes with Him. Your body and cycle are wonderfully made.

Sometimes I have the best conversations with my family during this time because I am extremely vulnerable in my feelings. We have also had huge blowout fights around this time, but the reconciliation is what makes our connections stronger.

This is what God wants for you: to be vulnerable with Him. Let Him know your feelings, your hurt, your struggles. He is there to listen (always), and He is steadfast.

A PRAYER

God, thank you for how we are beautifully made to be vulnerable. It is a gift to show others our feelings. We know that You are always there to listen to us in the heaviest of times. You are our rock when we need stability. Thank you for being there always. Amen.

Day 27

> What do you think? If a man owns a hundred sheep,
> and one of them wanders away,
> will he not leave the ninety-nine on the hills
> and go to look for the one that wandered off?
>
> —Matthew 18:12 (NIV)

I was lost—maybe not in a cult, but definitely drifting in the New Age. It all felt so harmless at first. I started with yoga, thinking I was just helping people feel better. Then came a few reiki sessions ... a crystal here and there ... and before I knew it, I had wandered far. But I didn't even realize it at the time. I had convinced myself that it was still "good."

You know what happened? Jesus came after me—again.

This time, He used people who were bold enough to speak truth into my life. They helped me see that I wasn't putting all my trust in Christ. I had one foot in the world and one in the Word.

When I read today's Scripture, I think of myself—the one sheep who strayed. But by His grace, I was brought back to the herd ... back to my Shepherd.

A PRAYER

Jesus, thank you for saving me when I wander. You are so steadfast and forgiving. Thank you for blessing my life and using those times I mess up as a testimony to Your forgiveness and love. Help me to find those that have also wandered and bring them back to You. Amen.

Day 28

I long to dwell in Your tent forever and take refuge in the shelter of Your wings.

—Psalm 61:4 (NIV)

I used to struggle with Premenstrual Syndrome (PMS), and, at one point, a conventional doctor diagnosed me with PMDD—Premenstrual Dysphoric Disorder, which is a more severe form of this complaint. I was prescribed birth control to "balance" my hormones and antidepressants to manage the side effects from the pills. This is far too common—and it rarely addresses the root cause.

I kept longing to be free from the symptoms, but I was looking in all the wrong places. It wasn't until I made a courageous decision to apply integrative medicine to my own health that my cycle began to heal—without medications. And more importantly, I realized that only the Lord can truly heal the soul. He is our true refuge. When we stop chasing fixes and start dwelling in Him, we find what we've been searching for all along.

He is seeking you—and He loves you more than you know.

A PRAYER

Jesus, You are always so perfect and graceful. Let us long to dwell in Your tent forever and take refuge in the shelter of Your wings. Give us the wisdom throughout the month to keep our eyes on You and commit our minds to Your words. We love You. In Jesus' name, Amen.

That's it, ladies. A month of daily devotionals to reflect on through your cycle. I pray the 28-Day Plan and Devotional give you clarity, encouragement, and hope as you take your next steps.

You may feel more vulnerable on certain days—and that's okay. We were created with these beautiful hormonal rhythms, and there is wisdom in leaning into them rather than resisting them.

When we stop fighting our emotions and start listening to them, we can respond with greater compassion, clarity, and purpose. These moments are welcome invitations to draw closer to God—to pause, reflect, and meditate on the gospel that grounds us in truth.

As you arrive at the end of the month, remember this: You can take refuge in the shelter of His wings (Psalm 91:4). He is steady, even when your emotions are not.

Some other things you can do that I have found helpful include:

- Play Christian music! Fill your home with positive music—it will elevate your mood. I even listen to Christian rap when I have a heavy weightlifting session. You decide what goes into your mind.
- Write out your favorite Scriptures and hang them in places around your home. For example, you can put them above your mirror while you are getting ready in the morning, on a cupboard door while you are cooking dinner, or in the mudroom to look at while putting on your shoes.

Spiritual warfare is real and active in the world around us, so it's essential to equip yourself with the sword of the Spirit—God's Word. Scripture strengthens, defends, and guides you. But don't stop there—learning how to care for your body through healthy, God-honoring changes will also empower you to become the strongest, most faithful version of yourself.

Conclusion

> Haven't I commanded you: be strong and courageous? Do not be afraid or discouraged, for the Lord your God is with you wherever you go.
>
> —Joshua 1:9 (CSB)

She thought she was following the right path spiritually and physically. And that walking down that road was best for her health. She took multiple supplements and peptides. Her environment was clean and her gut health perfected. Despite everything she was doing to remain healthy, something felt off. It was spiritual: She was practicing yoga and carrying around crystals, yet she still felt lost. All the sauna and cold plunging couldn't detox her from the windows she had opened. After deliverance, repentance and setting her eyes back on Jesus, she felt peace again.

This woman was me. I know that our spiritual health is connected to our physical health, but for some reason doctors don't like to talk about it. We are doing a disservice to our patients, and we are not serving our God either.

One of the biggest things that impacts women's health is one word. STRESS. It can be stress from viruses, an imbalanced gut microbiome, a moldy environment, or just emotional stress.

Your parents are aging. You're raising a child with special needs. Your boss is difficult, your neighbors seem cold, and now—even your dog has an illness. Life feels relentless. And honestly, it doesn't stop. Stress won't magically disappear. You can't eliminate every burden.

But you can give them to Jesus.

You can surrender the weight you're carrying and allow Him to carry it for you.

You can choose to embrace the sanctification process—letting the pressure form something beautiful in you, like olives crushed into pure, fragrant oil.

You may not be able to change your circumstances, but you can choose how you walk through them: with trust, perspective, and purpose.

> Therefore, since we are surrounded by such a great cloud of witnesses, let us throw off everything that hinders and the sin that so easily entangles. And let us run with perseverance the race marked out for us, fixing our eyes on Jesus, the pioneer and perfecter of faith. For the joy set before him he endured the cross, scorning its shame, and sat down at the right hand of the throne of God.
>
> —Hebrews 12: 1–2 (NIV)

I encourage you to continue using the tips and resources I've shared with you throughout this book. With God's help, you can be mindful of what you take in. As you lean on His strength, He will deepen your faith and sharpen your discernment to talk in truth.

This is a race of endurance—for your physical health and your spiritual growth. When distractions come (and they will), open your Bible and realign your heart with the faith-filled path God has for your health journey.

Remember, many physical struggles are rooted in spiritual ones.

Be diligent. Be strong and courageous. Be a light to other women walking through perimenopause.

Thank you for being brave, for doing the hard things, and for showing up in this season. I'm praying for you all.

To your healing and His glory,

Dr. Jen

Acknowledgments

Writing *The Perimenopause Reset* has been both a personal and professional journey—one that wouldn't have been possible without the unwavering support and grace of so many.

First, I thank Jesus Christ, the great Physician of both body and soul, and the sovereign Lord over every season of life. My desire in writing this book is to bring Him glory and to encourage women to view their health through the lens of Scripture.

To my mom and dad—thank you for always believing in me, encouraging me to pursue my calling as a physician, and for the countless phone calls filled with wisdom, support, and love. Your steady presence gave me the foundation to follow this path with purpose.

To my husband, Chip—thank you for always saying "yes." Yes to continued education, to fighting for patients, and to supporting this mission even when it meant sacrificing time or investing more to grow a vision that seeks to change the way we view health. Your belief in me means everything.

To my children—Anna, Declan, Cyrus, and Emery—I love you with my whole heart. Thank you for your encouragement, your patience, and your joy through the many hours I spent writing. You inspire me every single day.

To my friends—thank you for standing beside me. Writing this book brought moments of spiritual warfare, and your prayers—past, present, and future—will always be a shield. Thank you for helping me put on the full armor of God.

To my mentors and colleagues in integrative and functional medicine—thank you for your collaboration, inspiration, and dedication to root-cause healing. A special thank-you to Dr. Pam Smith, whose wisdom and leadership continue to shape and strengthen my work.

To my incredible team at Healthy by Dr. Jen—thank you for being part of this mission to restore health from the inside out. Your passion and excellence bring this vision to life every day.

And to every woman navigating perimenopause—thank you for your courage, your questions, and your trust. You are not alone, and your body can heal.

With all my gratitude,
Dr. Jen, Jenny, Mom

Dr. Jen

References and Resources

Chapter 1

Carneiro MF, Grotto D, Batista BL. Thyroid hormone disruption and neurotoxicity by mercury: Evidence from experimental and clinical studies. *Environ Res.* 2014;134:303-315.

Darbre PD, Harvey PW. Paraben esters: Review of recent studies of endocrine toxicity, absorption, esterase, and human exposure, and discussion of potential human health risks. *J Appl Toxicol.* 2008;28(5):561-578.

Desvergne B, Feige JN, Casals-Casas C. PPAR-mediated activity of phthalates: A link to the obesity epidemic? *Mol Cell Endocrinol.* 2009;304(1-2):43-48.

Diamanti-Kandarakis E, Bourguignon JP, Giudice LC, et al. Endocrine-disrupting chemicals: An Endocrine Society scientific statement. *Endocr Rev.* 2009;30(4):293-342. https://doi.org/10.1210/er.2009-0002

Grün F, Blumberg B. Endocrine disrupters as obesogens. *Mol Cell Endocrinol.* 2009;304(1-2):19-29. DOI: 10.1016/j.mce.2009.02.018

Jin Y, Lu Z, Chen Q. Endocrine-disrupting effects of heavy metals on thyroid hormones. *Environ Sci Pollut Res.* 2022;29(4):5041-5053.

Kabir ER, Rahman MS, Rahman I. A review on endocrine disruptors and their possible impacts on human health. *Environ Toxicol Pharmacol.* 2015;40(1):241-258.

Matsuda S. Bisphenol A causes hyperactivity in the male mouse by increasing dopaminergic activity. *Neuropharmacology.* 2010;59(1-2):97-104.

Meeker JD, Rossano MG, Protas B, et al. Environmental exposure to metals and male reproductive hormones: Circulating testosterone is inversely associated with blood cadmium and lead levels in men. *Reprod Toxicol.* 2009;27(2):137-142. DOI: 10.1016/j.fertnstert.2008.09.044

Richter CA, Birnbaum LS, Farabollini F, et al. In vivo effects of Bisphenol A in laboratory rodent studies. *Reprod Toxicol.* 2007;24(2):199-224. DOI: 10.1016/j.reprotox.2007.06.004

Rubin BS. Bisphenol A: An endocrine disruptor with widespread exposure and multiple effects. *J Steroid Biochem Mol Biol.* 2011;127(1-2):27-34. DOI: 10.1016/j.jsbmb.2011.05.002

Swan SH. Environmental phthalate exposure in relation to reproductive outcomes and other health endpoints in humans. *Environ Res.* 2008;108(2):177-184. DOI: 10.1016/j.envres.2008.08.007

Xu X, et al. Perinatal exposure to bisphenol A enhances anxiety and depression-like behaviors associated with alterations of estrogen receptor expression in the hippocampus of male mice. *J Psychiatr Res.* 2015;64:48-59.

Chapter 2

Darbre PD, Harvey PW. Paraben esters: Review of recent studies of endocrine toxicity, absorption, esterase, and human exposure, and discussion of potential human health risks. *J Appl Toxicol.* 2008;28(5):561-578.

Environmental Protection Agency (EPA). Basic Information about Lead in Drinking Water. EPA; 2018. Accessed from EPA.gov.

Fujii Y. Human exposure to endocrine-disrupting chemicals through daily use of personal care products. *Environ Sci Technol.* 2005;39(8):2978-2985.

Liu G. The legacy and emerging contaminants in non-stick cookware. *Environ Res.* 2020;184:109318.

Rogers MA. Impact of processed food on the human microbiome. *Nutrients.* 2020;12(1):45.

Steinemann A. Fragranced consumer products: exposures and effects from emissions. *Air Qual Atmos Health.* 2017;10(1):1-8.

Vandenberg LN, Hauser R, Marcus M, et al. Human exposure to bisphenol A (BPA). *Reprod Toxicol.* 2007;24(2):139-177. DOI: 10.1016/j.reprotox.2007.07.010

Wolkoff P. Indoor air pollutants in office environments: Assessment of comfort, health, and performance. *Int J Hyg Environ Health.* 2013;216(4):371-394.

Zock JP. Household cleaning products, irritant inhalation, and chronic respiratory symptoms. *Occup Environ Med.* 2007;64(3):165-170.

Chapter 3

Arora S, Singh S, Piazza GA, et al. Honokiol: A novel natural agent for cancer prevention and therapy. *Curr Mol Med.* 2012;12(10):1244-1252. doi:10.2174/156652412803833508

Dai X, Xie L, Liu K, et al. The neuropharmacological effects of magnolol and honokiol: A review of signal pathways and molecular mechanisms. *Curr Mol Pharmacol.* 2023;16(2):161-177. doi:10.2174/1874467215666220223141101

Hidese S, Ota M, Wakabayashi C, et al. Effects of chronic l-theanine administration in patients with major depressive disorder: An open-label study. *Acta Neuropsychiatr.* 2017;29(2):72-79. doi:10.1017/neu.2016.33

Hidese S, Ogawa S, Ota M, et al. Effects of L-theanine administration on stress-related symptoms and cognitive functions in healthy adults: A randomized controlled trial. *Nutrients.* 2019;11(10):2362. doi:10.3390/nu11102362

Hoilat GJ, Altowairqi AK, Ayas MF, et al. Larazotide acetate for treatment of celiac disease: A systematic review and meta-analysis of randomized controlled trials. *Clin Res Hepatol Gastroenterol.* 2022 Jan;46(1):101782. doi: 10.1016/j.clinre.2021.101782. Epub 2021 Jul 31. PMID: 34339872.

International Agency for Research on Cancer (IARC). IARC Monographs Volume 124: Night Shift Work. Accessed at: https://www.iarc.who.int/news-events/iarc-monographs-volume-124-night-shift-work/

Lin Y, Li Y, Zeng Y, et al. Pharmacology, toxicity, bioavailability, and formulation of magnolol: An update. *Front Pharmacol.* 2021;12:632767. doi:10.3389/fphar.2021.632767

Liu B, Hattori N, Nan-Yang Z, et al. Anxiolytic agent, dihydrohonokiol-B, recovers amyloid beta protein-induced neurotoxicity in cultured rat hippocampal neurons. *Neurosci Lett.* 2005;384(1-2):44-47. doi:10.1016/j.neulet.2005.04.081

Shen JL, Man KM, Huang PH, et al. Honokiol and magnolol as multifunctional antioxidative molecules for dermatologic disorders. *Molecules.* 2010;15(9):6452-6465. doi:10.3390/molecules15096452

White DJ, de Klerk S, Woods W, et al. Anti-stress, behavioural and magnetoencephalography effects of an L-theanine-based nutrient drink: A randomised, double-blind, placebo-controlled, crossover trial. *Nutrients.* 2016;8(1):53. doi:10.3390/nu8010053

Woodbury A, Yu SP, Wei L, et al. Neuro-modulating effects of honokiol: A review. *Front Neurol.* 2013;4:130. doi:10.3389/fneur.2013.00130

Zhang Y, Papantoniou K. Night shift work and its carcinogenicity. *Lancet Oncol.* 2019;20(10):E550. doi:10.1016/S1470-2045(19)30578-9

Chapter 4

Bakus C, Budge KL, Feigenblum N, et al. The impact of contraceptives on the vaginal microbiome in the non-pregnant state. *Front Microbiomes.* 2023.

Brabaharan S, Veettil SK, Kaiser JE, et al. Association of hormonal contraceptive use with adverse health outcomes: An umbrella review of meta-analyses of randomized clinical trials and cohort studies. *JAMA Netw Open.* 2022;5(1):e2143730. https://doi.org/10.1001/jamanetworkopen.2021.43730

Chang VC, Andreotti G, Ospina M, et al. Glyphosate exposure and urinary oxidative stress biomarkers in the Agricultural Health Study. *J Natl Cancer Inst.* 2023;115(4):394-404. https://doi.org/10.1093/jnci/djac242

Farrow A, Hull MGR, Northstone K, et al. Prolonged use of oral contraception before a planned pregnancy is associated with a decreased risk of delayed conception. *Hum Reprod.* 2002;17(10):2754-2761. https://doi.org/10.1093/humrep/17.10.2754

Goldner WS, Sandler DP, Yu F, et al. Pesticide use and thyroid disease among women in the Agricultural Health Study. *Am J Epidemiol.* 2010;171(4):455-464. https://doi.org/10.1093/aje/kwp404

Lammers KM, Lu R, Brownley J, et al. Gliadin induces an increase in intestinal permeability and zonulin release by binding to the chemokine receptor CXCR3. *Gastroenterology.* 2008;135(1):194-204.e3. https://doi.org/10.1053/j.gastro.2008.03.023

Thongprakaisang S, Thiantanawat A, Rangkadilok N, et al. Glyphosate induces human breast cancer cells growth via estrogen receptors. *Food Chem Toxicol.* 2013;59:129-136. https://doi.org/10.1016/j.fct.2013.05.057

Tucker J, Fischer T, Upjohn L, et al. Unapproved pharmaceutical ingredients included in dietary supplements associated with US Food and Drug Administration warnings. *JAMA Netw Open.* 2018;1(6):e183337. https://doi.org/10.1001/jamanetworkopen.2018.3337

Yonis H, Løkkegaard E, Kragholm K, et al. Stroke and myocardial infarction with contemporary hormonal contraception: Real-world, nationwide, prospective cohort study. *BMJ.* 2025;388:e082801. https://doi.org/10.1136/bmj-2024-082801

Chapter 5

Anton SD, Moehl K, Donahoo WT, et al. Flipping the metabolic switch: Understanding and applying the health benefits of fasting. *Obesity (Silver Spring)*. 2018;26(2):254-268. doi:10.1002/oby.22065

Bi Z, Wang L, Wang W. Evaluating the effects of glucagon-like peptide-1 receptor agonists on cognitive function in Alzheimer's disease: A systematic review and meta-analysis. *Adv Clin Exp Med*. 2023;32(11):1223–1231. doi:10.17219/acem/161734

Clifton S, Bryant S. Fasting and female hormone cycles: a review of current evidence. *Nutr Rev*. 2020.

De Giorgi R, Ghenciulescu A, Dziwisz O, et al. An analysis on the role of glucagon-like peptide-1 receptor agonists in cognitive and mental health disorders. *Nat. Mental Health* 3, 354–373 (2025). https://doi.org/10.1038/s44220-025-00390-x

Gillespie KA. Impact of time-restricted feeding on cortisol and metabolic health. *Clin Endocrinol*. 2022.

Hirota Y. Estrogen enhances insulin sensitivity through nuclear receptor pathways. *Endocrinology*. 2018.

Hoddy KK, Marlatt KL, Çetinkaya H, Ravussin E. Intermittent fasting and metabolic health: From religious fast to time-restricted feeding. *Obesity (Silver Spring)*. 2020;28(Suppl 1):S29-S37. doi:10.1002/oby.22829

Hutchison AT, Liu B, Wood RE, et al. Effects of intermittent versus continuous energy intakes on insulin sensitivity and metabolic risk in women with overweight. *Obesity (Silver Spring)*. 2019;27(1):50-58. doi:10.1002/oby.22345

Liu S, Zeng M, Wan W, Huang M, et al. The health-promoting effects and the mechanism of intermittent fasting. *J Diabetes Res*. 2023 Mar 3;2023:4038546. doi: 10.1155/2023/4038546. PMID: 36911497; PMCID: PMC10005873.

Lynch KE, et al. Intermittent fasting improves glucose metabolism and reduces oxidative stress in PCOS. *J Womens Health*. 2021.

Mandal S, Simmons N, Awan S, et al. Intermittent fasting: Eating by the clock for health and exercise performance. *BMJ Open Sport Exerc Med*. 2022 Jan 7;8(1):e001206. doi: 10.1136/bmjsem-2021-001206. PMID: 35070352; PMCID: PMC8744103

Morales-Suarez-Varela M, Collado Sánchez E, Peraita-Costa I, et al. Intermittent fasting and the possible benefits in obesity, diabetes, and multiple sclerosis: A systematic review of randomized clinical trials. *Nutrients*. 2021 Sep 13;13(9):3179. doi: 10.3390/nu13093179. PMID: 34579056; PMCID: PMC8469355.

Nina R, Huang L, Li Q, et al. Association of coffee consumption pattern and metabolic syndrome among middle-aged and older adults: A cross-sectional study. *Front Public Health*. 2023;11. https://doi.org/10.3389/fpubh.2023.1022616

Petersen MC, Shulman GI. Mechanisms of insulin action and insulin resistance. *Physiol Rev*. 2018;98(4):2133-2223. https://doi.org/10.1152/physrev.00063.2017

Perry RJ, Samuel VT, Petersen KF, Shulman GI. Mechanisms by which insulin stimulates hepatic glucose production in insulin-resistant states. *Cell Metab*. 2014;20(5):682-692. https://doi.org/10.1016/j.cmet.2014.09.021

Słuczanowska-Głąbowska S, Laszczyńska M, Piotrowska K, et al. Caloric restriction increases ratio of estrogen to androgen receptors expression in murine ovaries: Potential therapeutic implications. *J Ovarian Res*. 2015;8:57. doi:10.1186/s13048-015-0185-8

Smith RE, Havel PJ. Effects of intermittent fasting on inflammation and metabolic syndrome. *Nat Rev Metab.* 2019.

Wedick N, Brennan A, Sun Q, et al. Effects of caffeinated and decaffeinated coffee on biological risk factors for type 2 diabetes: A randomized controlled trial. *Nutr J.* 2011;10(1). https://doi.org/10.1186/1475-2891-10-93

Yarmolinsky J, Mueller N, Duncan B, et al. Coffee consumption, newly diagnosed diabetes, and other alterations in glucose homeostasis: A cross-sectional analysis of the longitudinal study of adult health (ELSA-Brasil). *PLoS One.* 2015;10(5):e0126469. https://doi.org/10.1371/journal.pone.0126469

CHAPTER 6

Araújo J, Cai J, Stevens J. Prevalence of optimal metabolic health in American adults: National health and nutrition examination survey 2009-2016. *Metab Syndr Relat Disord.* 2019 Feb;17(1):46-52. doi: 10.1089/met.2018.0105. Epub 2018 Nov 27. PMID: 30484738.

Azemati B, Rajaram S, Jaceldo-Siegl K, et al. Animal-protein intake is associated with insulin raesistance in Adventist Health Study 2 (AHS-2) calibration substudy participants: A cross-sectional analysis. *Curr Dev Nutr.* 2017;1(4):e000299. https://doi.org/10.3945/cdn.116.000299

Blatt A, Roe L, Rolls B. Increasing the protein content of meals and its effect on daily energy intake. *J Am Diet Assoc.* 2011;111(2):290-294. https://doi.org/10.1016/j.jada.2010.10.047

Del Río JP, Alliende M, Molina N, et al. Steroid hormones and their action in women's brains: The importance of hormonal balance. *Front Public Health.* 2018;6. https://doi.org/10.3389/fpubh.2018.00141

Diep CA, Daniel A, Mauro LJ, et al. Estrogen receptor beta signaling in the regulation of ERα-positive breast cancer. *J Mol Endocrinol.* 2015;54(2). https://doi.org/10.1530/JME-14-0252

Dighriri IM, Alsubaie AM, Hakami FM, et al. Effects of omega-3 polyunsaturated fatty acids on brain functions: A systematic review. *Cureus.* 2022;14(10):e30091. https://doi.org/10.7759/cureus.30091

Gök V. Effect of replacing beef fat with poppy seed oil on quality of Turkish sucuk. *Korean J Food Sci Anim Resour.* 2015;35(2):240-247. https://doi.org/10.5851/kosfa.2015.35.2.240

Gutiérrez S, Svahn SL, Johansson ME. Effects of omega-3 fatty acids on immune cells. *Int J Mol Sci.* 2019;20(20):5028. https://doi.org/10.3390/ijms20205028

Kerr A, Hart L, Davis H, et al. Improved strength recovery and reduced fatigue with suppressed plasma myostatin following supplementation of a vicia faba hydrolysate, in a healthy male population. *Nutrients.* 2023;15(4):986. https://doi.org/10.3390/nu15040986

Khor B, Tallman D, Karupaiah T, et al. Nutritional adequacy of animal-based and plant-based Asian diets for chronic kidney disease patients: A modeling study. *Nutrients.* 2021;13(10):3341. https://doi.org/10.3390/nu13103341

Lombardo M, Rizzo G, Feraco A, et al. High plant-based diet and physical activity in women during menopausal transition. *Nutr Food Sci.* 2021;52(3):547-560. https://doi.org/10.1108/nfs-06-2021-0195

Luger M, Schindler K, Kruschitz R, Ludvik B. Feasibility and efficacy of an isocaloric high-protein vs. standard diet on insulin requirement, body weight, and metabolic parameters in patients with type 2 diabetes on insulin therapy. *Exp Clin Endocrinol Diabetes.* 2013;121(05):286-294. https://doi.org/10.1055/s-0033-1341472

Mohammed H, Russell IA, Stark R, et al. Progesterone receptor modulates ERα action in breast cancer. *Nature.* 2015;523(7560):313-317. https://doi.org/10.1038/nature14583

Moloudpour B, Jam S, Darbandi M, et al. Association of plant-based diet and estimated glomerular filtration rate in Iranian Kurdish population: The RANCD cohort study. *Res Sq.* 2022. https://doi.org/10.21203/rs.3.rs-1843740/v1

Pasiakos S, Agarwal S, Lieberman H, Fulgoni V. Sources and amounts of animal, dairy, and plant protein intake of U.S. adults in 2007–2010. *Nutrients.* 2015;7(8):7058-7069. https://doi.org/10.3390/nu7085322

Pawluk AR, Sumler D. BPC-157: A novel therapeutic for tissue repair and gut health. *Adv Exp Med Biol.* 2015;856:213–227.

Peppiatt MJ, Edwards CM, Oliver JR. GLP-1 receptor agonists in the management of obesity and metabolic syndrome. *J Endocrinol.* 2022;252(1):R29–R44.

Ribeiro R. Rapid benefits in older age from transition to whole food diet regardless of protein source or fat to carbohydrate ratio: A randomized control trial. *Aging Cell.* 2024;23(11). https://doi.org/10.1111/acel.14276

Różańska MB, Kowalczewski PŁ, Tomaszewska-Gras J, Dwiecki K, Mildner–Sandkühler JF. Cold-pressed rapeseed oil: Processing effects on oxidative stability. *BMC Med.* 2023;21:440. https://doi.org/10.1186/s12916-023-03146-5

Shoskes DA, Gittelman M. KPV as an anti-inflammatory peptide for skin and gut health. *Int J Pept Res Ther.* 2020;26(4):1637–1644.

Smith J, Kassem M. Peptides for muscle preservation: Emerging roles of PeptiStrong in aging. *Clin Interv Aging.* 2019;14:785–793.

Szkudlarz S. Seed-roasting process affects oxidative stability of cold-pressed oils. *Antioxidants.* 2019;8(8):313. https://doi.org/10.3390/antiox8080313

Tucker L, Erickson A, LeCheminant J, et al. Dairy consumption and insulin resistance: The role of body fat, physical activity, and energy intake. *J Diabetes Res.* 2015;2015:206959. https://doi.org/10.1155/2015/206959

Wojcik J, Devassy J, Wu Y, et al. Protein source in a high-protein diet modulates reductions in insulin resistance and hepatic steatosis in fa/fa Zucker rats. *Obesity.* 2016;24(1):123-131. https://doi.org/10.1002/oby.21312

Yu K, Huang Z, Xu X, et al. Estrogen receptor function: Impact on the human endometrium. *Front Endocrinol (Lausanne).* 2022;13:827724. https://doi.org/10.3389/fendo.2022.827724

Zeng Y, Li S, Xiong G, Wan J. Influences of protein to energy ratios in breakfast on mood, alertness, and attention in the healthy undergraduate students. *Health.* 2011;3(6):383-393. https://doi.org/10.4236/health.2011.36065

CHAPTER 7

Aliyari H, Golabi S, Sahraei H, et al. Perceived stress and cognition function quantification in a scary video game: An electroencephalogram features and biochemical measures. *Basic Clin Neurosci J.* 2023;14(2):297-310. https://doi.org/10.32598/bcn.2022.3811.1

Beghini F, Pullman J, Alexander M, et al. Gut microbiome strain-sharing within isolated village social networks. *Nature.* 2025;637:167–175. https://doi.org/10.1038/s41586-024-08222-

Chang X, Jiang X, Mkandarwire T, et al. Associations between adverse childhood experiences and health outcomes in adults aged 18–59 years. *PLoS One.* 2019;14(2):e0211850. https://doi.org/10.1371/journal.pone.0211850

Fredrickson BL. The role of positive emotions in positive psychology: The broaden-and-build theory of positive emotions. *Am Psychol.* 2001;56(3):218-226. https://doi.org/10.1037/0003-066x.56.3.218

Gaviria J, Rey G, Bolton TB, et al. Dynamic functional brain networks underlying the temporal inertia of negative emotions. *bioRxiv.* Preprint. Published March 26, 2021. https://doi.org/10.1101/2021.03.26.437275

Giano Z, Wheeler DL, Hubach RD. The frequencies and disparities of adverse childhood experiences in the U.S. *BMC Public Health.* 2020;20:1327. https://doi.org/10.1186/s12889-020-09411-z

Qiao-Tasserit E, Quesada MG, Antico L, et al. Transient emotional events and individual affective traits affect emotion recognition in a perceptual decision-making task. *PLoS One.* 2017;12(2):e0171375. https://doi.org/10.1371/journal.pone.0171375

Senaratne DNS, Thakkar B, Smith BH, et al. The impact of adverse childhood experiences on multimorbidity: A systematic review and meta-analysis. *BMC Med.* 2024;22:315. https://doi.org/10.1186/s12916-024-03505-w

CHAPTER 8

Csala B, Springinsfeld CM, Köteles F. The relationship between yoga and spirituality: A systematic review of empirical research. *Front Psychol.* 2021;12:695939. doi:10.3389/fpsyg.2021.695939

Duraimani S. A cross-sectional and longitudinal study of the effects of a mindfulness meditation mobile application platform on reducing stress and anxiety. *Int J Yoga.* 2019;12(3):226. doi:10.4103/ijoy.ijoy_56_18

Hatmalyakin D, Utami Y, Wihastuti T. The effect of mindfulness meditation on mental illness among nurse in ICU and ICCU. *Res J Life Sci.* 2019;6(1):66-71. doi:10.21776/ub.rjls.2019.006.01.8

Pace T, Negi L, Sivilli T, et al. Innate immune, neuroendocrine, and behavioral responses to psychosocial stress do not predict subsequent compassion meditation practice time. *Psychoneuroendocrinology.* 2010;35(2):310-315. doi:10.1016/j.psyneuen.2009.06.008

Prasanna Venkatesh L, Vandhana S. Insights on Surya Namaskar from its origin to application towards health. *J Ayurveda Integr Med.* 2022;13(2):100530. doi:10.1016/j.jaim.2021.10.002

Sadowski A, Wexler R, Hanes D, et al. Meditative practices, stress, and sleep among students studying complementary and integrative health: A cross-sectional analysis. *BMC Complement Med Ther*. 2022;22(1). doi:10.1186/s12906-022-03582-5

Walker A. "God is my doctor": Mindfulness meditation/prayer as a spiritual well-being coping strategy for Jamaican school principals to manage their work-related stress and anxiety. *J Educ Adm*. 2020;58(4):467-480. doi:10.1108/jea-06-2019-0097

Chapter 10

Aslam M, Shauket R, Yousaf Z, et al. Nutraceutical intervention of seeds in the treatment of polycystic ovarian syndrome: A systematic review. *Pakistan BioMedical Journal*. 2021;4(2):281–286. https://doi.org/10.54393/pbmj.v4i2.100

Barlow A, Blodgett J, Williams S, et al. Injury incidence, severity, and type across the menstrual cycle in elite female professional footballers: A prospective three-season cohort study. https://doi.org/10.1101/2023.07.12.23292497

Benton M, Hutchins A, Dawes J. Effect of menstrual cycle on resting metabolism: A systematic review and meta-analysis. *Plos One*. 2020;15(7):e0236025. https://doi.org/10.1371/journal.pone.0236025

Brown S, Jiang B, McElwee-Malloy M, et al. Fluctuations of hyperglycemia and insulin sensitivity are linked to menstrual cycle phases in women with t1d. *Journal of Diabetes Science and Technology*. 2015;9(6):1192-1199. https://doi.org/10.1177/1932296815608400

Dey S, Dasgupta D, Roy S. Blood glucose levels at two different phases of menstrual cycle: A study on a group of Bengali-speaking Hindu ethnic populations of West Bengal, India. *The Oriental Anthropologist, a Bi-Annual International Journal of the Science of Man*. 2019;19(1):55-63. https://doi.org/10.1177/0972558x19835371

Écochard R, Bouchard T, Leiva R, et al. Characterization of hormonal profiles during the luteal phase in regularly menstruating women. *Fertility and Sterility*, 2017;108(1), 175-182.e1. https://doi.org/10.1016/j.fertnstert.2017.05.012

Evans S, Levin F. Response to alcohol in women: Role of the menstrual cycle and a family history of alcoholism. *Drug and Alcohol Dependence*. 2011;114(1):18-30. https://doi.org/10.1016/j.drugalcdep.2010.09.001

Galasinska K, Szymkow A. Enhanced originality of ideas in women during ovulation: A within-subject design study. *Front Psychol*. 2022;13:859108. doi:10.3389/fpsyg.2022.859108. PMID: 35756251; PMCID: PMC9222335.

Galasinska K, Szymkow A. The more fertile, the more creative: Changes in women's creative potential across the ovulatory cycle. *Int J Environ Res Public Health*. 2021;18(10):5390. doi:10.3390/ijerph18105390. PMID: 34070114; PMCID: PMC8158362.

Garner TB, Hester JM, Carothers A, Diaz FJ. Role of zinc in female reproduction. Biol Reprod. 2021 May 7;104(5):976-994. doi: 10.1093/biolre/ioab023. PMID: 33598687; PMCID: PMC8599883.

Génolini C. Characterization of hormonal profiles during the luteal phase in regularly menstruating women. *Fertility and Sterility*. 2017;108(1):175-182.e1. https://doi.org/10.1016/j.fertnstert.2017.05.012

Haggans CJ, Hutchins AM, Olson BA, Thomas W, Martini MC, Slavin JL. Effect of flaxseed consumption on urinary estrogen metabolites in postmenopausal women. *Nutr Cancer*. 1999;33(2):188-95. doi: 10.1207/S15327914NC330211. PMID: 10368815.

Haggans CJ, Travelli EJ, Thomas W, Martini MC, Slavin JL. The effect of flaxseed and wheat bran consumption on urinary estrogen metabolites in premenopausal women. *Cancer Epidemiol Biomarkers Prev*. 2000 Jul;9(7):719-25. PMID: 10919743.

Hanzawa F, Nomura S, Sakuma E, Uchida T, Ikeda S. Dietary sesame seed and its lignan, sesamin, increase tocopherol and phylloquinone concentrations in male rats. *J Nutr*. 2013 Jul;143(7):1067-73. doi: 10.3945/jn.113.176636. Epub 2013 May 22. PMID: 23700348.

Higuchi T, Ueno T, Uchiyama S, Matsuki S, Ogawa M, Takamatsu K. Effect of γ-tocopherol supplementation on premenstrual symptoms and natriuresis: A randomized, double-blind, placebo-controlled study. *BMC Complement Med Ther*. 2023 Apr 28; 23(1):136. doi:10.1186/s12906-023-03962-5.

Hummel J, Benkendorff C, Fritsche L, et al. Brain insulin action on peripheral insulin sensitivity in women depends on menstrual cycle phase. *Nat Metab*. 2023 Sep;5(9):1475-1482. doi: 10.1038/s42255-023-00869-w. Epub 2023 Sep 21. PMID: 37735274; PMCID: PMC10513929.

Irfan T, Seher K, Rizwan B, et al. Role of Seed Cycling in Polycystic Ovaries Syndrome. *Pakistan BioMedical Journal*. 2021;4(2). https://doi.org/10.54393/pbmj.v4i2.122

Kamal-Eldin, Afaf & Moazzami, Ali & Washi, Sidiga. (2011). Sesame Seed Lignans: Potent Physiological Modulators and Possible Ingredients in Functional Foods & Nutraceuticals. Recent patents on food, nutrition & agriculture. 3. 17-29. 10.2174/2212798411103010017.

Kulzhanova D, Turesheva A, Donayeva A, et al. The cortisol levels in the follicular and luteal phases of the healthy menstruating women: A meta-analysis. *Eur Rev Med Pharmacol Sci*. 2023;27(17):8171-8179. doi:10.26355/eurrev_202309_33577. PMID: 37750645.

Md Amin NA, Sheikh Abdul Kadir SH, Arshad AH, Abdul Aziz N, Abdul Nasir NA, Ab Latip N. Are Vitamin E Supplementation Beneficial for Female Gynaecology Health and Diseases? *Molecules*. 2022; 27(6):1896. https://doi.org/10.3390/molecules27061896

Miyamoto M. Exploring the relationship between nutritional intake and menstrual cycle in elite female athletes. *Peerj*. 2023;11:e16108. https://doi.org/10.7717/peerj.16108

Nowak J, Podsiadło A, Hudzik B, et al. Food intake changes across the menstrual cycle: A preliminary study. *Nursing and Public Health*. 2020;10(1):5-11. https://doi.org/10.17219/pzp/114280

Okazaki M, Kaneko M, Ishida Y, et al. Changes in the width of the tibiofibular syndesmosis related to lower extremity joint dynamics and neuromuscular coordination on drop landing during the menstrual cycle. *Orthopaedic Journal of Sports Medicine*. 2017;5(9). https://doi.org/10.1177/2325967117724753

Salem A. Variation of leptin during menstrual cycle and its relation to the hypothalamic–pituitary–gonadal (hpg) axis: A systematic review. *International Journal of Women S Health*. 2021;13:445-458. https://doi.org/10.2147/ijwh.s309299

Sawai A, Tochigi Y, Kavaliova N, et al. MRI reveals menstrually-related muscle edema that negatively affects athletic agility in young women. *Plos One*, 13(1), e0191022. https://doi.org/10.1371/journal.pone.0191022

Shi Y, Xiao S, Wang C, et al. Effect of nutrition on plasma lipid profile and mRNA levels of ovarian genes involved in steroid hormone synthesis in hu sheep during luteal phase1. *Journal of Animal Science*. 2013;91(11):5229-5239. https://doi.org/10.2527/jas.2013-6450

Sims S, Kerksick C, Smith-Ryan A, et al. International society of sports nutrition position stand: Nutritional concerns of the female athlete. *Journal of the International Society of Sports Nutrition*. 2023;20(1). https://doi.org/10.1080/15502783.2023.2204066

Tada Y, Yoshizaki T, Tomata Y, et al. The impact of menstrual cycle phases on cardiac autonomic nervous system activity: An observational study considering lifestyle (diet, physical activity, and sleep) among female college students. *Journal of Nutritional Science and Vitaminology*. 2017;63(4):249-255. https://doi.org/10.3177/jnsv.63.249

Wagner R, Kullmann S, Heni M. Brain insulin action on peripheral insulin sensitivity in women depends on menstrual cycle phase. *Nat Metab*. 2023;5(9):1475-1482. doi:10.1038/s42255-023-00869-w. PMID: 37735274; PMCID: PMC10513929.

Wunderle K, Hoeger K, Wasserman E, Bazarian J. Menstrual phase as predictor of outcome after mild traumatic brain injury in women. *Journal of Head Trauma Rehabilitation*. 2014;29(5):E1-E8. https://doi.org/10.1097/htr.0000000000000006

Wu WH, Kang YP, Wang NH, Jou HJ, Wang TA. Sesame ingestion affects sex hormones, antioxidant status, and blood lipids in postmenopausal women. *J Nutr*. 2006 May;136(5):1270-5. doi: 10.1093/jn/136.5.1270. PMID: 16614415.

Wyskida K, Franik G, Wikarek T, Owczarek A, et al. The levels of adipokines in relation to hormonal changes during the menstrual cycle in young, normal-weight women. *Endocrine Connections*. 2017;6(8):892-900. https://doi.org/10.1530/ec-17-0186

Zarei S, Mosalanejad L, Ghobadifar M. Blood glucose levels, insulin concentrations, and insulin resistance in healthy women and women with premenstrual syndrome: a comparative study. *Clinical and Experimental Reproductive Medicine*. 2013;40(2):76. https://doi.org/10.5653/cerm.2013.40.2.76

Resources

Website

https://www.healthybydrjen.com/

YouTube

https://www.youtube.com/@integrativedrmom

Social Media Sites

https://www.instagram.com/integrativedrmom/
https://www.facebook.com/IntegrativeDrMom
https://x.com/integrativedrma

Podcast

The Integrative Health Podcast with Dr. Jen
https://open.spotify.com/show/3noyG8FGUirxkmpBpyAm2O
https://theintegrativehealthpodcast.buzzsprout.com
https://podcasts.apple.com/us/podcast/the-integrative-health-podcast-with-dr-jen/id1541507452

Product Recommendations

https://www.healthybydrjen.com/drjenfavorites
https://www.amazon.com/shop/integrativedrmom
https://healthybydrjen.shop/

INDEX

B

Bible study, 127, 139, 141, 145-147, 154-156, 192, 194, 201, 203, 208, 214
Bisphenol A (BPA); plastics and hormone disruption, 16, 18-19, 23
Body-spirit connection, 141

C

Circadian rhythm, 28-29, 31-32, 43
    optimizing hormones with, 92, 09, 125
    sleep-wake cycles and, 28, 29, 31, 32
Cleanse
    body (nutrition, detoxification), 7, 51, 83, 99, 103, 105, 115, 125, 172, 175
    environment (home toxins, air quality), 15, 16, 26, 51, 61, 131, 132, 138, 139, 140, 178
    spirit (emotional release, negativity), 137-138
Connect
    with faith, 140
    with healthier products, 21
    with hormonal signals, 3, 37, 73-75, 84, 96, 98-99, 103, 107
Continuous glucose monitors (CGM), 73, 82-83, 87, 89, 94, 168, 180
Cultivate
    a healthy habitat, 26, 33-34, 39, 61, 95, 98, 111, 115, 149, 153
    muscle strength, 90
    sleep environment, 42

D

Detoxification
    liver detox, 67, 69, 71, 114, 120
    gentle detox practices, 72
DHEA, 9, 11, 55, 96-98, 102, 111, 113-114, 124

E

Endocrine disruptors, 17, 20, 55
    household sources of, 23, 137, 200
    effects on hormones, 17, 20, 55
Environmental toxins, 54
Estrogen, 5-6, 29, 34-35, 49, 56, 62-64, 66,-67, 78, 96, 100-101, 114, 168, 222-224
    cycle and fluctuations, 19, 39, 92, 98, 109, 111, 113, 123, 147, 164, 168-169, 173
    estrogen dominance, 6, 35-36, 64-65, 67-68, 78, 99, 111, 113

F

Faith-based living, 3, 132, 140, 154, 179
Fasting, 74, 76, 78, 79, 94, 172, 186, 222
    intermittent fasting benefits, 73-79
    blood sugar and fasting, 73-79

G

GMO crops and hormone health, 52
Gluten and intestinal permeability, 57
Gut-hormone axis, 55

H

Heavy metals and hormone disruption, 54
Hormonal shifts, 125
   changes in perimenopause, 82, 103, 110, 228
   strategies to support balance, 65

I

Integrative medicine, benefits of, 132

L

Liver detoxification, 67, 69, 71, 114, 120
Lifestyle changes
   exercise, 15, 30, 40, 82, 87, 89, 99, 103-104, 136, 163, 169, 172-173, 222
   nutrition, 7, 51, 83, 99, 103, 105, 115, 125, 172, 175
   stress reduction, 145

M

Meditation and breathwork (Christian perspective), 145
Menstrual cycle, 5
   cycle syncing for diet and exercise, 163
Mold exposure, 34, 38
   prevention and remediation, 38
Mycotoxins, 34-37

N

Nutrition in perimenopause, 7, 51, 99, 103, 105, 115, 125, 175, 223, 227, 228
   balancing macronutrients, 29
   reducing sugar, 19

P

Parabens, effects of, 17, 23, 24
Peptides, 7, 91, 122-123, 125, 224
   GLP-1, 91, 92, 93, 106, 123, 224
   KPV, BPC-157, 123
Perimenopause, 5-6, 12, 36, 55, 57, 90-92, 98, 101, 103, 105-106, 108-109, 111, 114, 122-123, 137, 145, 163, 217
   common symptoms, 4
   hormonal changes in, 82, 103, 110, 228
Phthalates, effects of, 17, 23
Plastics and hormone health
Progesterone, 6, 44, 49, 79, 97-99, 101-102, 112-114, 164, 168, 224

S

Sleep hygiene
   circadian rhythm and, 28-29, 31-32, 43
   smart supplementation for, 43
Spiritual life
   Christ-centered approach, 142
   spiritual warfare, 127-129, 162, 185, 217

T

Testosterone, changes in, 6, 49
Toxins
   environmental, 54
   in household products, 23, 137, 200

V

Vagus nerve, 148, 149, 152
Vitamins and supplements for perimenopause, 114

Y

Yoga
   Christian discernment of, 144, 225

About the Author

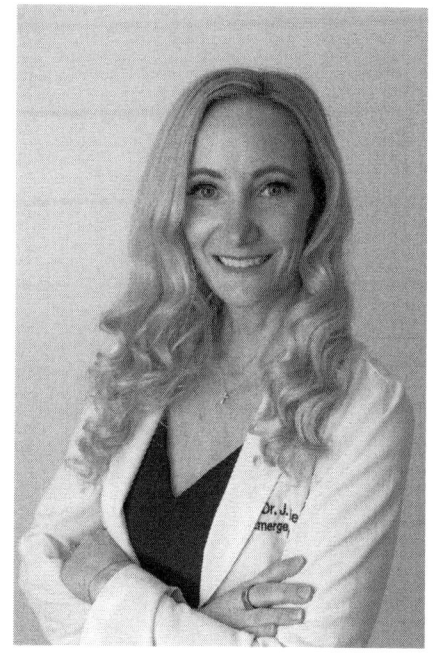

Dr. Jen Pfleghaar is a double board-certified physician in Emergency Medicine and Integrative Medicine. She earned her medical degree from the Lake Erie College of Osteopathic Medicine, completed her residency at St. Vincent's Mercy Hospital, and pursued fellowship training at the prestigious Andrew Weil Center for Integrative Medicine.

With over 20 years of experience, Dr. Jen blends clinical expertise with a passion for root-cause healing. She is the co-author of *Eat. Sleep. Move. Breathe.*, a practical guide to healthy living, and proudly serves on the board of the Invisible Disabilities Association. She is also a member of the American Osteopathic Association's Bureau of Osteopathic Research and Public Health. A sought-after national speaker, Dr. Jen is known for her engaging talks on integrative medicine, hormone health, and whole-body wellness.

Her journey into integrative medicine began after a personal diagnosis of Hashimoto's thyroiditis—a pivotal moment that inspired her to explore autoimmune disease, hormone balance, and holistic wellness. Now in remission, she dedicates her practice to helping others find healing in body, mind, and spirit.

Beyond her medical work, Dr. Jen is a devoted wife and proud mom of four. She lives with her family on a mini farm in Tennessee, where she raises backyard chickens, lifts weights, and finds daily strength and purpose through her faith in God and the truth of Scripture, especially her favorite book, the Bible. She shares education and encouragement on Instagram and YouTube as @integrativedrmom and leads her wellness community at healthybydrjen.com.

Printed in Dunstable, United Kingdom